PATHOLOGICAL SELF-CRITICISM

ASSESSMENT AND TREATMENT

THE PLENUM SERIES IN SOCIAL/CLINICAL PSYCHOLOGY
Series Editor: C. R. Snyder
University of Kansas
Lawrence, Kansas

PATHOLOGICAL SELF-CRITICISM

ASSESSMENT AND TREATMENT

RAYMOND M. BERGNER

Illinois State University
Normal, Illinois

PLENUM PRESS • NEW YORK AND LONDON

Library of Congress Cataloging-in-Publication Data

On file

ISBN 0-306-44961-7

©1995 Plenum Press, New York
A Division of Plenum Publishing Corporation
233 Spring Street, New York, N.Y. 10013

10 9 8 7 6 5 4 3 2 1

PREFACE

Countless therapy clients fail repeatedly to criticize themselves in ways that are constructive and beneficial. Instead, they resort to self-critical practices that not only fail to produce their intended results but also prove quite injurious. In many cases, the extent of this injury is so great that the practices may be considered pathological. That is, they engender very significant restrictions in the ability of these persons to participate in life in meaningful and fulfilling ways. To borrow a phrase from Freud, these practices severely damage their ability "to love and to work."

A few brief observations may serve to illustrate the widespread prevalence of such pathological self-criticism. Not only do many clients present it as a problem in its own right ("I'm incredibly hard on myself," "I'm extremely perfectionistic," etc.) but also it is often at the root of other quite prevalent clinical compliants and conditions. For example, many clients report that they suffer from "low self-esteem." Upon inspection, it may be seen that a person's self-esteem is essentially that person's summary appraisal of his or her own worth or value (Ossorio, 1982). As such, it is clearly and directly a product of how the individual is functioning as a critic of himself or herself (McKay & Fanning, 1992). Second, and closely related, numerous clients report extreme senses of ineligibility for valued things in life. They perceive themselves to be not good enough to interest the desired partner, competent enough to land the attractive job, or talented enough to merit coveted opportunities in artistic, athletic, or other arenas. Like self-esteem, exaggerated perceptions of ineligibility, and the behavioral restrictions that follow from them, have their basis in judgmental behaviors that individuals have enacted as critics of themselves. To cite a third and final example, it is worth noting that most established theories of the etiology of depression hold that maladaptive self-criticism is deeply implicated in this condition. Cognitive investigators report that depressed persons have an extremely "negative view of self . . . as inadequate, deserted, and worthless" (Beck & Weishaar, 1989, p. 296). Learned helplessness theorists observe that the depressed, as critics of themselves, are prone to attribute negative events to factors that are within themselves, are global, and are unchangeable, resulting in strong feelings of personal helplessness (Peterson, Maier, & Seligman, 1993). Psychoanalysts testify that depressed individuals are enormously self-deprecating and hateful toward themselves (Freud, 1917/1958; Rubin, 1975). In one way or another, all of these theorists are making the same general contention: persons become depressed in good part because they subject themselves to highly injurious self-critical actions.

The foregoing examples of connections between maladaptive self-criticism and other common clinical problems are but the tip of the iceberg. In the chapters that follow, many further connections will be documented. These include links to such problems as being extremely vulnerable to the criticisms of others, experiencing difficulties with regulating one's own behavior, living one's life excessivley preoccupied with what others think, and being unable to diagnose and change one's own problematic behavioral tendencies. In the end, a portrait emerges of pathological self-criticism as highly prevalent and as profound in its implications for individuals' lives.

A BRIEF OUTLINE

In this volume, the problem of pathological self-criticism will be approached in the following ways. In the first four chapters of the book, which are primarily concerned with clarifying the phenomena and with assessment, (1) the most commonly observed patterns of maladaptive criticism will be described and their consequences noted, and (2) a number of means for assessing these patterns and the factors that are maintaining them will be related. In the remainder of the book, which is concerned with treatment; (3) a set of therapeutic interventions will be provided for helping clients to abandon pathological self-critical practices in favor of more constructive ones; (4) some effective responses to common resistances that clients present will be related; and (5) a therapeutic relationship that greatly enhances the efficacy of all of the other interventions mentioned throughout the book will be described.

NATURE OF THE PRESENT WORK

The clinical descriptions and interventions detailed in this book derive from a number of sources. Their origins lie in the research, theoretical, and practical literature in clinical and social psychology, and in countless contributions from colleagues, supervisors, and conference presenters over the course of the last 25 years. In the end, however, all of these "inputs" have been subjected to clinical trial and evaluation by the author in his own therapeutic work with pathologically self-critical persons. The ideas presented in this book represent a distillation of the most illuminating and, above all, *effective* approaches that resulted from this process.

INTENDED AUDIENCE

The present volume is intended for several audiences. The first is psychotherapists who are currently in practice or in training. The second is researchers and theoreticians in clinical and social psychology with an interest in topics such as cognitive-behavioral therapy, social cognition, self-attribution, self-control therapy, and etiological factors in mental disorders. The third and final audience is lay persons who have an interest in matters of self-criticism. While the book is not a self-help volume, its numerous case illustrations, pragmatic conceptualizations, and procedural recommendations should be of considerable value to those wishing to alter their own destructive self-critical practices.

ACKNOWLEDGMENTS

I am greatly indebted to four individuals for their contributions to the book. First, I wish to thank Cynthia Good Mojab for her very extensive assistance in doing the research, in discussing many of its ideas with me, in copyediting, and in serving as the coauthor of Chapter 4. Second, I wish to thank my wife, Laurie Bergner, who initially gave me the idea for this book, provided a considerable number of ideas and observations based on her own clinical cases, and helped immeasurably with the copyediting. Third, I wish to thank my series editor, Dr. C. R. Snyder, for alerting me to numerous helpful links between my own work and that of others, for editing the final manuscript, and for being so enthusiastically supportive of the entire project. Finally, I wish to express my gratitude to my mentor, Peter Ossorio, for giving me the intellectual background that made this book a possibility.

CONTENTS

Chapter 5

Helping Clients to Abandon Pathological
Self-Critical Practices 67

Chapter 9

Chapter 10

PATHOLOGICAL SELF-CRITICISM

ASSESSMENT AND TREATMENT

CHAPTER 1

THE PROBLEM OF PATHOLOGICAL SELF-CRITICISM
AN OVERVIEW

Every man is a suffering-machine and happiness-machine combined. ... Sometimes, a man's make-up and disposition are such that his misery-machine is able to do all of the business.

MARK TWAIN, *The Mysterious Stranger*

The subject of this book is self-criticism. Its central idea is that how persons exercise the role of critic with respect to themselves has enormous consequences for their personal happiness and for the quality of their lives. Unfortunately, countless individuals, including many who seek psychotherapeutic help, have learned to criticize themselves in ways that are highly destructive (Driscoll, 1981, 1989; McKay & Fanning, 1992; Rubin, 1975). This book is devoted to the therapeutic betterment of these individuals.

WHAT IS PATHOLOGICAL SELF-CRITICISM?

In general, criticism is a social practice whose point is to benefit the person criticized. When the English teacher criticizes the student's essay, the parent appraises the child's behavior, or the coach evaluates the athlete's technique, it is generally understood that such criticism should be beneficial to those receiving it. It should in-

1

form them, for example, that their behavior is successful or unsuccessful, what there is about the behavior that accounts for its success or lack thereof, and/or how the behavior might be improved in the future. When criticism fails this understood requirement, it is typically regarded as defective. We say that it was not "constructive," not "helpful," "ineffective because it did not give its recipient any ideas about how to change," and the like.

With this general requirement in mind, a very important and fundamental question may be posed of any given criticism that an individual might render toward himself or herself: Does this criticism enhance the ability of this person to participate in life in meaningful and fulfilling ways or is it destructive of such ability? Does it, for example, increase the individual's ability to have full and satisfying relationships, to immerse him- or herself in meaningful work, or to pursue other life interests successfully and enjoyably? When the answer to such questions is in the affirmative, the criticism may be regarded as constructive. When the answer is negative—that the criticism is damaging to the individual's ability to participate fully and meaningfully—it may be regarded as destructive. In cases where this damage is very significant, such as those that will constitute the primary focus of this book, we may speak of "pathological" self-criticism (see Ossorio, 1985, on the concept of pathology).

In the chapters to follow, an extensive look will be taken at different types of such pathological self-criticism. At this point, in order to become better oriented to this notion, let us take a brief, preliminary look at some clients who practice such self-criticism, and at some of the general consequences that frequently befall them.

David, a 42-year-old history teacher, generally works hard all day, is highly productive, and makes substantial inroads on his valued "things-to-do" list. However, when he sits down at night to watch television, he invariably poisons his leisure time with the following sorts of self-recriminations: "What am I doing sitting here watching this mindless drivel; I'm lazy, unproductive, sitting around like a bum when there are important things I really should be doing." (In response to therapist query) "I did work hard all day, but so what? That's yesterday's news; that's done and over with; you can't live your life dwelling on yesterday's glories."

After the breakup of an important relationship, Karen, a 35-year-old social worker, becomes deeply depressed and self-hating. Despite abundant evidence that her former partner's fears of commitment were decisive to the breakup, she appraises herself and her role in the following ways: "Somehow, even though I can't say how, I believe that I screwed this relationship up. I do believe it when you (therapist) say that he is afraid of commitment, but I can't stop feeling like there must be something wrong with me—something just not good enough about me.... It just feels like I'm unlovable ... like every time I let a guy really know me, he ends up leaving me."

Finally, Alex, a 29-year-old accountant who entered therapy after being hospitalized for depression, relates the following: "I'm self-critical, and I'm critical of others, and I think it helps me. I'm hard on myself, not willing to accept second best or to tolerate faults. I don't compare myself to ordinary people but to the best. For example, where my tennis game is concerned, I compare myself to the Wimbledon champion. I always pale in comparison and I feel inadequate, but there's nothing worse than settling for average. You know those movie critics who give two thumbs up for good movies and two thumbs down for bad ones? Well, I never give two thumbs up for anything I do. But, I give a lot of two thumbs down."

In these self-critical scenarios, it is hard to find much that is constructive. We see individuals branding themselves with degrading labels such as "unlovable," "lazy," "bum," and "defective" ("something wrong with me"). In doing so, they are interpreting their perceived failures, not as tolerable and perhaps alterable human mistakes, but as proof positive that they are characterologically defective, disqualified sorts of persons. Further, we see them being strongly committed to impossible standards that doom them to failure in their own eyes: they must be as good as the best in all areas of life or be productive 24 hours a day. We see them failing to make the punishment fit the crime or, in many cases, the supposed crime—blistering themselves for sitting down to watch television after a hard day's work or degrading themselves mercilessly for their supposed personal failure in a romantic relationship. We see them recognizing and acknowledging only failures and weaknesses but dismissing strengths, efforts, and accomplishments. They are always ready with "two thumbs down" but never with "two thumbs up."

Some Consequences of Pathological Self-Criticism

There are generally some benefits or advantages that derive from habitually treating oneself in such ways (Driscoll, 1981, 1984;

McKay & Fanning, 1992). For example, some persons may be able to "put the screws to themselves" and thereby goad themselves to high levels of productivity for a period of time (Ossorio, 1976). However, such treatment is almost invariably a relatively ineffective means for securing such benefits and is always on balance damaging to individuals. The costs of pathological self-criticism vastly outweigh its benefits. Some of the most common and important of these costs, all of which will be discussed at length in later chapters follow.

Damaged Self-Esteem

A person's self-esteem is that person's summary appraisal of his or her own worth or goodness. As such, it is clearly and directly a product of the individual's functioning as a critic of self (McKay & Fanning, 1992). Others may hold an individual in high or low esteem, but it is the esteem in which persons hold themselves, by definition, that is self-esteem. If they repeatedly brand themselves "unlovable," "selfish," "screwed-up," and the like; repeatedly declare themselves miserable failures for not living up to impossible standards; repeatedly attack themselves in hateful, abusive ways; or engage in other injurious critical practices, their self-esteem will be abysmal.

Personal Ineligibility

When persons appraise themselves destructively, they are doing something far more consequential than merely (as some clients put it) "beating themselves up." They are also making evaluations that profoundly affect their sense of eligibility to behave in the world (Bergner, 1987, 1988). For example, if they appraise themselves as "unlovable," this is just another way of saying that they are ineligible to be loved; if "stupid," that they are ineligible for the myriad things in life that call for intelligence; if "insignificant nothings," that they are ineligible to have relationships with the worthy "somethings" of the world. Appraising themselves so, they will typically experience tremendous doubt, despair, and/or behavioral paralysis in their pursuit of desired relationships, jobs, and other life opportunities.

Negative Emotional States

When individuals engage repeatedly in such actions as branding themselves with degrading labels, declaring themselves ineligible, and judging themselves failures vis-à-vis impossible standards, they are likely to be *depressed* (Beck, Rush, Shaw, & Emery, 1979; Bergner, 1983, 1988). When they appraise themselves in such a way that important situations they must confront seem beyond their ability to manage, they will be *anxious* (Beck & Emery, 1985; Bergner, 1983; Kelly, 1955). When they judge themselves the bearers of highly stigmatizing, socially discrediting characteristics, they will experience shame (Bergner, 1983; Goffman, 1963). When they repeatedly evaluate themselves as morally deficient and blameworthy, they will experience *guilt* (Bergner, 1983; Ossorio, 1976). When they appraise themselves as helpless to alter negative life circumstances, they will experience *hopelessness and despair* (Bergner, 1983; Peterson, Maier, & Seligman, 1993). In these and other ways, destructive self-criticism will culminate in negative emotional states.

Vulnerability to Others' Criticisms

Pathological self-criticism frequently renders individuals excessively vulnerable to the criticisms of others in a number of important ways. First, believing the worst about themselves, they will be all too ready to concur immediately with the negative judgments of others (McKay & Fanning, 1992; Stone & Stone, 1993): "They must be right; if they find me lacking, I must *be* lacking." Second, because they esteem themselves so little, they will tend to become excessively dependent on the reception of esteem from others in forms such as approval, love, and recognition (Stone & Stone, 1993). Third and finally, being so fearful of the negative opinions of others and so desperate for their approval, pathologically self-critical persons will tend to adapt their behavior inappropriately to what they perceive to be others' desires. Confronted with decisions about what action to take, they do not ask themselves "What do my personal principles and/or desires indicate?" Rather, their paramount concern becomes "What will they think?"

Dismissal of Positives

When persons are always prepared to pounce critically upon their mistakes and faults but never to recognize their strengths, efforts, and accomplishments, they rob themselves of crucial knowledge and satisfactions in life. Such individuals might, for example, get a positive evaluation at work, be pursued romantically by an attractive other, or complete a difficult project in a quality fashion. When unacknowledged or discounted by the person, however, such events will have little or no positive impact on their sense of personal efficacy (Bandura, 1982, 1992), desirability, or moral decency. Further, such events will result at best in meager feelings of joy, accomplishment, or satisfaction. Overall, in these self-critical scenarios, a great deal of punishment but very little reward, is evident.

Inability to Change

Finally, one hallmark of pathological self-criticism is that, even when it represents a response to truly problematic actions or characteristics, it contains little that the person rendering it might use to change his or her behavior in the future. If one examines the quotations above, denunciatory labels, impositions of impossible standards, and harsh prosecutorial attacks abound. But there is little in the way of useful problem diagnoses or of implementable prescriptions for change. The situation is entirely analogous to one where a teacher might respond to a student's mistake by saying, "You are so stupid," rather than by saying, "Terry, I think the absence of good topic sentences and headings is what's hurting the organization in your essays. Next time, why don't you...."

OBSTACLES TO CHANGING
PATHOLOGICAL SELF-CRITICISM

In the face of so much pain and so many destructive consequences, one would think that people would readily abandon pathological self-critical practices. However, clinical observation reveals both that this is not the case and that there are many important obstacles to individuals doing so. While these obstacles will be discussed at length in later chapters (see especially Chapters 4 and 8), a brief review of them here will begin to convey the difficulties destructively self-critical persons face in their attempts to change.

Many individuals engage in destructively self-critical acts in such a habitual, reflexive fashion that they cannot observe what they are doing to themselves (cf. Beck & Weishaar, 1989; Haaga & Beck, 1992, on "automatic thoughts"). Like many other appraisals in life (e.g., a grammatical one that I should say "me" rather than "I" in a certain sentence), the appraisals of self are instantaneous, highly automatic, and occur largely outside of awareness. Obviously, it is rather difficult to alter what one cannot observe.

A second major reason why it is so difficult to alter destructive self-critical practices is that most persons who employ them feel powerless to do so. When they cannot observe what they are doing, their whole sense will be that their misery is visited upon them by sources beyond their control (Bergner, 1993). Even when they are able to observe their own self-critical acts, they often report a sense that they are not in control of these. Rather, it appears to them that "the critic" has a life of its own. It seems to be a voice inside them but not really "them" and not subject to their decisions. When the destructive self-criticism is long-standing, as it almost always is in clinical populations, the sense of powerlessness will be deepened: "I have been doing this all my life; it's so ingrained, so habitual; how can I ever stop?"

A third reason why self-critical patterns are difficult to change is that those who employ them often have strong investments in maintaining them. "If I gave up my insistence on perfection, I would be settling for mediocrity, and that is completely unaccept-able to me." "If I don't use very strong and severe measures to deal with myself, I'll never change; being a more benign critic to myself seems like a weak, ineffectual 'slap on the wrist.'" "I'm afraid I'd become conceited and egotistical if I started to appraise myself in more positive ways, and I would hate to become that sort of per-son." The list goes on and on. But the basic point remains that de-structive self-critical acts, when one examines them closely, are pur-posive acts (Driscoll, 1981, 1989). People engage in them to accomplish important purposes in their lives, and they are not ready to give them up as long as they believe that doing so would mean relinquishing the accomplishment of these purposes.

PURPOSE OF THIS BOOK

In pathological self-criticism, then, we have a problem that is extremely common, that is ruinous to the lives and happiness of people, and that entails significant obstacles to change. Despite what might seem at this point a gloomy and imposing picture, however, pathological self-criticism can be treated successfully and in some cases in a surprisingly short period of time. The primary purpose of this book is to set forth a comprehensive set of therapeu-tic conceptualizations, ideas, and strategies that the author has found highly effective for the accomplishment of this objective.

The therapeutic approaches described in this book have de-rived from many sources: the theoretical and research literatures in clinical and social psychology; contributions over the years from teachers, supervisors, and colleagues; and personal experimentation and observation in treatment situations. They have been gathered over the course of some 25 years of clinical work, and might be said to have survived the long struggle of the survival of the fittest, since along the way many other approaches have been tried and found insufficiently effective. The "survivors" presented in this book are those that have proven most effective in helping individuals to abandon pathological self-critical practices and to adopt and commit themselves to far more effective, humane, and constructive alternatives.

OVERVIEW OF BOOK

This book is organized as follows. In Chapters 2 and 3, the most common and important pathological self-critical patterns presented by clients, as well as their typical consequences, are described. In Chapter 4, the focus shifts to clinical assessment of these patterns and includes an extended section devoted to origins, functions, and other causal factors in need of such assessment. In Chapter 5, a therapeutic strategy designed to enable individuals to abandon maladaptive self-critical practices is presented. In Chapter 6, a positive conception of self-criticism, one that details a far more humane, effective, and constructive approach to this task, is advanced. In Chapter 7, therapeutic procedures for helping individuals to acquire and adopt this more constructive approach are related. In Chapter 8, the most frequently encountered resistances and obstacles that clients present, as well as numerous therapeutic responses to counter these effectively, will be discussed. In Chapter 9, a positive therapeutic relationship that greatly enhances the efficacy of all of the other approaches described in this book is articulated. Finally, in Chapter 10, some concluding considerations are offered.

PRIVATE
SELF-DEGRADATION
CEREMONIES

I would really like to go over there and have lunch with that
little red-haired girl, but (sigh!) I can't, because I'm a nothing
and she's a something.

Charlie Brown (Shulz, 1968)

Shannon, a 20-year-old college senior, reported at her intake session
that she continued to suffer repercussions from an event that had occurred many years previously. While in the eighth grade at a
parochial school, her class had held a graduation party at a state
park. During the party, a boy to whom she was strongly attracted
asked her to walk with him alone in the forest. In the course of their
walk, the boy suddenly thrust his hand into her pants and touched
her vaginal area. Shocked, confused, and in some measure not wanting to displease the boy, Shannon froze. Before she could recover and
say or do anything (a period she estimated at perhaps five seconds),
the boy removed his hand. Nothing further transpired between the
two. As a result of this single, brief incident, Shannon branded herself a "slut," and with this, radically reassessed her entire social position. In her eyes, she had "fallen" from being sexually whole, good,
and valuable to being "easy," "dirty," and sexually devalued. She believed that she could no longer presume to have a place among the
valued "nice boys and girls" in her peer group, but must regard herself a stigmatized outcast. As a result, she withdrew socially and experienced an extremely lonely and painful adolescence.

9

Jim, a teacher in his forties, reported a dream in which he found himself at a party at the home of an old friend. Again and again at this party, people greeted him but then quickly excused themselves on flimsy pretexts, and left him alone. He awoke, rather sad, thinking, "I really am very unimportant and insignificant to others. I have no place in their lives. If it were not for my wife, I doubt that anyone would seek me out socially, and I really think it's largely because, truth be known, deep down I don't really care about people." These self-criticisms duplicated ones that he rendered frequently in everyday life. As a consequence of his alleged lack of caring, he experienced considerable guilt and a sense of personal deficiency—of "something basically human being missing in me." As a consequence of his perceived unimportance to others, he found it quite difficult, among other things, to be assertive with them; when he did so (usually somewhat haltingly and apologetically), he was visited by a sense that he was "imposing" on them in a way that would provoke their resentment.

Marcy, a 22-year-old recent college graduate, made an ill-advised statement in the course of a job interview. Upon recognizing her mistake, she thought to herself, "I'm so incredibly stupid; will I ever stop saying the wrong thing?" This self-characterization, "stupid," was one of several that her parents had employed repeatedly while she was growing up (others included "selfish," "lazy," and "emotionally unstable"). She had learned to apply it reflexively to herself whenever she made a mistake or encountered failure, and it carried a depth of painful meaning for her befitting all those years of being so characterized. When seen in therapy several days after the job interview, Marcy remained quite preoccupied with this incident and very distraught over the reconfirmation of her inadequacy that she perceived in it.

In all of these cases, we observe a common theme. Like Charlie Brown in the opening quote, Shannon, Jim, and Marcy criticize themselves in a certain characteristic way. In reaction to perceived transgressions, mistakes, failures, and weaknesses, they brand themselves with highly invidious, disqualifying labels such as "stupid," "insignificant," "uncaring," "slut," and "nothing." Unlike many others who might utter similar self-accusations in a moment of pique but not really mean them, these individuals stand deeply and fully behind their indictments. The effects of such critic acts, particularly when persons stamp in the same destructive labels time after time and year after year, can be extremely devastating to them. A helpful concept for capturing the precise nature of this devastation is one formulated many years ago by Garfinkel (1957), that of a "degradation ceremony."

THE CONCEPT OF A DEGRADATION CEREMONY

Harold Garfinkel, in his 1957 sociological classic, "Conditions of Successful Degradation Ceremonies," first articulated the concept of a "degradation ceremony." The concept has been employed heavily since that time by Descriptive Psychologists (e.g., Bergner, 1993; Ossorio, 1976, 1978; Schwartz, 1979) in their accounts of psychopathological phenomena. The paradigm cases of degradation ceremonies are formal public rituals in which the place or *status* of an individual in some community is drastically diminished or even eliminated. Examples of such rituals include court martials, rites of excommunication, and impeachment hearings. The essence of these ceremonies is that the individual in question, for reasons bearing on his or her (allegedly) discreditable conduct, is publicly declared to be "no longer one of us"—no longer a member in good standing of the community. In lesser cases (e.g., demotions), he or she is declared to be still a member of the community, but one of diminished status. Unless the individual can find some way to effectively refuse these denunciations, he or she is rendered no longer *eligible* to participate in the community in question in the same way as before, and perhaps not at all.

By way of illustration, consider the hypothetical case of a lieutenant in the military who has been found guilty of a grave breach of his military duties. One morning, his company is assembled on the parade grounds and he is brought before them. The company commander steps forward, faces the lieutenant, and before everyone makes a formal announcement to the effect that the lieutenant has engaged in conduct unbecoming an officer. Further, the commander proclaims, this conduct is deemed a reflection of the lieutenant's character and reveals him to have been all along unfit to be an officer. In light of these things, the commander strips the lieutenant of his rank and demotes him to the rank of private (from Ossorio, 1976).

The basic force of this ceremony is that the lieutenant is literally "de-graded." That is, he is removed from one grade or status in his community and relocated to another, diminished one

(Garfinkel, 1957). The essential difference that this relocation makes is that the new status conveys drastic reductions in his eligibilities to participate in his community. Where once he could give orders to most of the men and women on the base, reside in special quarters, and in general enjoy a wide range of officers' privileges, he now can do none of these. His community status, and with it his behavioral eligibilities, have been radically diminished (Bergner, 1987, 1988, 1990: Ossorio, 1976, 1978).

PRIVATE SELF-DEGRADATION CEREMONIES

In the paradigm case just presented, one person formally degrades another before witnesses. In the derivative case known as a private self-degradation ceremony (Ossorio, 1976, 1978), one person informally enacts all three roles: he or she serves as denouncer, as denounced, and as witness. This individual privately declares himself or herself to be a certain sort of degraded person (e.g., a "slut," a "selfish, loveless narcissist," an "idiot," or an "emotionally unstable person"). With such self-degradation come many of the same kinds of consequences detailed in the example, and more. In the following section, let us take a closer look at the precise nature of these consequences.

CONSEQUENCES OF SELF-DEGRADATION

PERSONAL INELIGIBILITY

When individuals subject themselves to significant self-degradation, they seriously erode their sense of personal eligibility to engage in the social practices of their communities. When Shannon, for example, declares herself a "slut," she simultaneously reassesses her eligibilities for relationships with others. With her self-reappraisal, she has in her own eyes fallen from being sexually pure and valuable to being sexually devalued. With this, she further believes herself disqualified from acceptance by "nice boys and girls" in her peer group and regards herself a stigmatized outcast. Her situation is precisely analogous to Charlie Brown's, who, deeming himself a "nothing," simultaneously appraises himself as ineligible for relationships with all "somethings" and, most importantly, with the much-desired little red-haired girl.

As noted briefly in Chapter 1, when persons appraise themselves as "unlovable," this is just another way of saying that they are ineligible to be loved; when "stupid," that they are ineligible for the myriad things in life that call for intelligence; when "mentally disturbed" (depending on the connotations this has for them), that they are ineligible to appraise realistically their circumstances and to render logical, well-grounded judgments and decisions—in other words, to behave competently at all. Their critic acts become essentially acts of self-disqualification. They are responding to things going wrong by declaring in effect that not only were they deficient on this occasion, but they are the kinds of persons who are disqualified from doing any better. By dint of the defective character or incompetence or moral blemish captured in their self-assigned labels, they mark themselves as persons who are ineligible or unable to succeed (cf. Goffman, 1963, on stigmatizing labels and how these serve to "spoil" whole identities).

BEHAVIORAL RESTRICTION

When people believe themselves to be disqualified, they tend to refrain from behavior relevant to the sphere of disqualification or to have great difficulty engaging in such behavior. Shannon, believing herself a "slut," withdrew from her classmates and declined all dates. Jim, appraising himself an insignificant cipher in others' lives, found it extraordinarily difficult to express his desires, to take strong stands with others, or to adopt anything but a pleasing, placating stance in his marriage and elsewhere (which provided him with ammunition for yet another painful self-characterization, that of "wimp"). Marcy, evaluating herself as intellectually incompetent, repeatedly quit jobs and discontinued tasks prematurely, believing they were beyond her abilities (see Bandura, 1982, 1992, on the behavioral consequences of self-efficacy beliefs).

Persons who have assigned highly degrading statuses to themselves also restrict their lives because they fear that if they took behavioral risks, they would be subjected to painful experiences that would only reconfirm their degraded status (McKay & Fanning, 1992). If they took chances and pursued desired relationships with others, they would be painfully rejected and their status as unattractive and inferior would be verified once again. If they went out on dates proposed by others, they would be treated as sexual objects, buttressing their suspicions that "that's all that men could possibly want from the likes of me." If they applied for a job, put in for a promotion, or submitted their work for publication, they would surely be rebuffed and their inadequacy reconfirmed. Thus, they conclude, it is far better to "pull in one's horns" and restrict one's life than it is to suffer such painful reconfirmations.

EMOTIONAL DISTRESS

Any scenario entailing a very negative critical appraisal of one's place in the world, a consequent belief that one is ineligible to pursue personally important and valued things in life, and an ultimate failure to act is bound to result in emotional distress. Shannon, saddled with her appraisal of herself as a slut, shut herself off from others and suffered an utterly miserable adolescence marked by shame and depression. Marcy, forever criticizing herself as stupid and incompetent, confronted many situations believing that she was "in over her head" and therefore sure to fail and suffered repeated bouts of anxiety. And, in our whimsical but psychologically accurate example, Charlie Brown, behaviorally paralyzed by his woeful estimation of his own place and eligibilities, sits, head down, sighing and depressed.

When labels assigned (e.g., "stupid" or "incompetent") are such that persons continually feel unable to succeed at vital tasks confronting them, the resulting emotional state will be *anxiety* (Beck & Emery, 1985; Bergner, 1983; Kelly, 1955). When labels are such that individuals believe themselves the bearers of socially discrediting, stigmatizing characteristics (e.g., "sexual deviant" or "mentally ill person"), the resulting emotional state will be *shame* (Bergner, 1983; Goffman, 1963; Ossorio, 1976). When labels have to do with moral deficiency (e.g., "selfish" or "unable to love"), the resulting emotional state will be *guilt* (Bergner, 1983; Ossorio, 1976). When labels capture conditions that permanently and hopelessly disqualify one (e.g., "born loser" or "intellectually inferior"), the resulting emotional states will tend to be *sadness and despair*, the emotions most characteristic of depressive states (Beck et al., 1979; Bergner, 1983, 1988; Ossorio, 1976). Finally, because these are not mutually exclusive appraisals, there will be degrading self-attributions (e.g., "stupid," "unable to love," or "sexual deviant") that will result in multiple negative emotions for their attributors.

LACK OF A PRESCRIPTION FOR CHANGE

When self-criticism consists of little more than the assignment of a degrading label, there is nothing prescriptive in the picture. The situation is entirely analogous to one in which a teacher would correct a student by saying, "You stupid idiot!" rather than by saying, "Look, Susie, here's the problem; you're not using your topic sentences and headings to alert your reader to what is to follow." In such a situation, there is first of all no usable problem formulation (diagnosis). Second, and consequently, there is no possibility of a recipe for corrective action that might result in more successful (and in some contexts, more responsible) behavior in the future. The entire critical episode comes to an end with the imposition of the degrading self-attribution, not with the creation of useful problem formulations and prescriptions that might enable the individual to improve matters.

HYPERSENSITIVITY TO OTHERS' CRITICISMS

"The truth hurts," an old aphorism has it. It is the degrading criticisms leveled by others that persons take to be the truth, or that they at least fear or suspect may be the truth, that devastate them the most (McKay & Fanning, 1992; Stone & Stone, 1993). Under conditions where individuals are rendering (or at least suspecting) the same indictments as those handed down by others and regarding these indictments as having global negative implications for their personal worth, they are most vulnerable to them. On the other hand, when individuals simply do not believe the "charges leveled against them" or do not believe that they constitute the "federal case" alleged by the other, they are far less vulnerable (cf. Snyder & Higgins, 1988; Snyder, Higgins, & Stucky, 1983, on the adaptive benefits of excuses in the face of negative input). In the latter case, the criticism may hurt them to some degree, but it does not have the power to devastate them—to create the awful sinking feeling that "They are right; I am that sort of deficient person" and the misery and preoccupation that come in its wake.

It is also those external criticisms that persons agree with that cause them to be hypersensitive in the second sense of that word. That is, they cause them to be "touchy"—to be prone in the face of criticism to counterattack immediately and to refuse to consider anything said by the other—because they must defend themselves at all costs from the sorts of hurt and degradation described above (McKay & Fanning, 1992; Stone & Stone, 1993). Again, if they at heart did not share the appraisal, they would have far less reason to be so touchy in the face of it.

Inability to Be the Final Arbiter of One's Own Status

Finally, there are certain labels or statuses that persons assign to themselves that leave them in an especially vulnerable position to be controlled by the beliefs of others about them. These statuses include ones such as "irrational," "intellectually inferior," and "mentally ill." All of these self-attributions involve a lack of belief in one's own competence at seeing the world realistically and deriving sound, logical judgments and decisions based on this. Where such faith in their ability to do so is lacking, individuals are left vulnerable to looking to others of supposedly greater realism and judgment when making appraisals of themselves.

For example, Marcy appraised herself as intellectually inferior and emotionally unstable. The daughter of a professional man of considerable intelligence and accomplishments, she related her typical reaction to his repeated harsh indictments of her: "When my father criticizes me, it's like God is speaking, and I just can't bring myself to believe anything other than what he is telling me." Marcy had disqualified herself as a competent and legitimate judge of her own place and value in the world and had placed these appraisals (and this fundamental power) in the hands of her father. She had become, in the phraseology of Marshall (1991, p. 262), a "non-self-status-assigner."

DEGRADING LABELS ARE
IMPERVIOUS TO CHANGE

Consider for a moment the hypothetical example of a politician who has come to be regarded by the press and the public as "a totally political animal, motivated solely by political expediency." Once such an attribution has become fixed in the public mind, no action by this politician, regardless of how selflessly or nobly motivated it might in fact be, need disconfirm it. Virtually anything he or she does may be seen by the public as "playing up to the constituents," "trying to shore up political support with group X," "trying to project a certain image to the electorate," and the like. The label has become immune to the ordinary sorts of empirical disconfirmation, and therefore potentially permanent.

In the same manner, once individuals brand themselves with degrading labels, in the face of contradictory evidence they tend not to alter the label but to assimilate new facts to it (Beck & Weishaar,

1989; Bergner, 1987; Ossorio, 1976, 1978). The upshot of this tendency is that such self-characterizations become locked in and highly resistant to change. For example, a young college woman, Sandy, had long appraised herself as "intellectually dull." She had acquired this view of herself in the context of being the youngest child in a family composed of rather accomplished individuals. Growing up, she was always a bit behind everyone else since she was two years younger than her next youngest sibling. The family treated her as the cute, amusing, but slightly dim "baby of the family," and she came to adopt such a view of herself. Sandy, however, had completed grade school with virtually all As and had matriculated from a very prestigious and competitive high school with a 3.5 grade point average. When she entered therapy, she was carrying the identical 3.5 average while taking a rather demanding curriculum at a large state university.

In the course of therapy, Sandy was asked how she squared all of the evidence from her scholastic career with her self-characterization as "intellectually dull." How could she continue to look at the countless As and Bs from teachers in demanding courses and still regard herself as unintelligent? In teasing out the answer to this question, Sandy revealed what amounted to unwitting discounting strategies that preserved her label in the face of disconfirmatory evidence. Confronted with an A, for example, her favorite explanation was along the lines of the old saying about genius being more a matter of perspiration than of inspiration: "Isn't it amazing what a dull person like me can do if I work hard enough!" On other occasions, she might tell herself that (1) she had been lucky, (2) the professor was not very demanding, (3) that she had fortunately studied just the right things, and/or (4) it was her roommate's help that got her through. Finally, when Sandy occasionally did receive a bad evaluation, she viewed this simply as confirmation of her low ability. The net result of these discounting strategies was that her self-assigned label of "intellectually dull" had remained remarkably intact despite massive evidence to the contrary.

RELEVANT OBSERVATIONS FROM OTHER THEORISTS

Other clinical investigators over the years have noted the phenomenon of self-assigned labels or statuses being impervious to empirical disconfirmation and have provided a number of clinically useful explanations for this phenomenon. In this section, several of the more important ones will be reviewed.

Beck and his associates (Beck et al., 1979; Beck & Weishaar, 1989) have reported relevant observations of persons with long and deeply held negative beliefs about themselves. These "self-schemas" might include personal convictions such as, "I am unlovable," "I am grossly incompetent," or "I am a completely selfish person." For individuals harboring such conceptions of themselves, their convictions will tend to serve a highly biasing function. When schema-related events occur in their lives, they will be prone to interpret these events as confirming their prior prejudice or schema about themselves. It is as if they reason that, "X is the bedrock, immutable, truth about me; it is simply a given; what has happened must therefore be consistent with X." In the process of drawing such conclusions, these persons will tend to make characteristic logical errors (e.g., overgeneralizing, magnifying or minimizing the significance of events, or drawing arbitrary inferences as to their significance) whose ultimate effect is to distort the meaning of the events in the direction of confirming the schematic beliefs. In this scenario, the schemata or self-labels determine the meaning of the facts; the facts do not determine the content of the labels. Ossorio earlier made essentially the same observation, and crystallized it in a helpful aphorism: "Status takes precedence over fact" (1976, p. 28).

Seligman and associates (Abramson, Seligman, & Teasdale, 1978; Nolen-Hoeksema, Girgus, & Seligman, 1987; Peterson et al., 1993) have demonstrated an "insidious attributional style" in persons prone to depression. In this style, negative events that befall the individual such as rejections or failures tend to be interpreted as due to factors that are internal to the individual (e.g., one's traits or abilities), global (i.e., affecting many aspects of one's life), and stable (permanent). Thus, for example, the loss of a job might be interpreted as due to one's personal incompetence. The second dimension of this attributional style is that positive events such as job offers, promotions, social invitations, or other successes are attributed to factors that are external to oneself, transitory, and situation-specific. Thus, for example, securing a good job offer might be attributed not to one's possession of the relevant competencies but to luck or even to the job interviewer's poor judgment. Such an attributional style clearly works to preserve degrading labels. Negative events merely confirm them, while positive events, because they are attributed to transient situational factors, never disprove or negate them.

Finally, Ossorio (1976) has discussed the phenomenon of "biased search." Here, persons tend to notice facts that are consistent with their self-assigned labels but not facts that are inconsistent with them. Thus, an individual who sees herself as "selfish" might notice and become distraught about an episode where she declines to help a friend, but she will barely register the countless other times when she gives to her family and friends. Again, the net result will be that her degrading label, "selfish," will remain intact despite the existence of numerous facts about herself that would seem to contradict it.

For all of these reasons, then, self-assigned degrading statuses tend over time to become the given, unquestioned, bedrock "truth." The critics who assign them become more and more prone to reflexly assimilate all new facts to them and less and less aware of the possibility of reconsidering them in light of discrepant empirical evidence. When certain clinical observers (e.g., Rubin, 1975) speak of these self-denigrating beliefs as being "unconscious" and as "operating more or less autonomously," I believe it is largely to the above sorts of facts that they are alluding.

DESTRUCTIVE SELF-DEGRADATION VERSUS CONSTRUCTIVE RECOGNITION OF PERSONAL LIMITS

Not every instance of self-criticism that results in the appraisal of diminished status and eligibility is problematic. For example, in the aftermath of a family crisis, an individual might draw the sober conclusion that "I really have been a very selfish person for quite a long time." Or, another individual, after pursuing physics as a college major for several years, might determine that "I'll never be a good physicist because, despite my best efforts, I don't have the ability to master the required mathematics."

What is different about such cases and the cases cited previously that been designated pathological? In both, there is the presence of disqualifying labels or self-attributions, so the difference cannot be anything so simple as the mere presence or absence of these.

In general, three criteria are helpful in making the distinction between destructive and constructive self-labeling. The first of these is realism versus lack of realism. Where the imposition of disqualifying labels seems discrepant with the available evidence, this would constitute grounds for regarding it as needlessly destructive.

The example cited above of Sandy, the young woman who appraised herself as intellectually deficient despite massive evidence to the contrary, is a very clear illustration of this.

A second criterion has to do with the wider implications drawn by persons criticizing themselves. For some persons, having the alleged deficiency captured in their labels constitutes grounds for regarding themselves as degraded, defective human beings. For them, their entire basic worth is thrown into question by their self-attribution. For other persons, there is no such implication. In effect, they seem to be saying, "Yes, I have this limitation and it's by no means a good thing, but it does not render me worthless." Needless to say, where the implications drawn are ones of global worthlessness, criticism is far more destructive.

A third and final criterion is the degree of self-punitiveness present. In some cases, what is observed is persons not only branding themselves with degrading labels but also in effect savaging themselves with scathing self-attacks. In more constructive cases, the note struck is more, "It's not a good thing; I am angry (guilty, disappointed, etc.) with myself; but beating myself into the ground about it is not going to help me go on and responsibly undertake the changes that I need to make."

SUMMARY

Summarizing what has been said to this point, when persons brand themselves with highly degrading labels, they create a host of problems. By dint of these self-characterizations, they cast themselves as ineligible for a wide variety of meaningful and rewarding forms of participation in life, behave consistently with this by restricting their lives, and suffer the emotional consequences of such self-degradation and restriction. Furthermore, the practice of employing these labels creates conditions that are antithetical to constructive change. They contain nothing in the form of useful problem formulations that might be used to generate prescriptions for improved or more responsible behavior, and they render the individual far more vulnerable to being devastated and even controlled by the criticisms of other persons. Finally, the degrading labels assigned tend for a variety of reasons to be impervious to being changed by contradictory evidence, and thus become crystallized into fixed, negative, unalterable beliefs about themselves.

In closing, it should be noted that all of these elements often result in the creation of destructive cycles in persons' lives (C. R. Snyder, personal communication, 1994). This is because the consequences of self-degradation typically provide individuals with further grounds for degrading themselves. An example of such a cycle occurred in the case of Jim, the teacher described above who appraised himself as highly insignificant to others. As a consequence of this self-appraisal, he would rarely "presume" to "impose on" others by asserting himself or by taking meaningful roles in their lives (e.g., visiting a bereaved acquaintance). In response to his behavior, others ignored him to a considerable degree or only engaged him socially in superficial ways. Perceiving this, Jim reconfirmed the validity of his "insignificant" label and also attributed other degrading statuses to himself such as "wimp" and "uncaring person" (cf. Rosenthal, 1974, on "self-fulfilling prophecies"). While the details will vary from case to case, such destructive cycles of self-degradation leading to negative consequences leading to further self-degradation, and so on, are the rule and not the exception.

CHAPTER 3

OTHER SELF-CRITICAL PATTERNS

In this chapter, three additional patterns of pathological self-criticism and their consequences will be described. These include (1) perfectionistic scenarios in which individuals employ humanly impossible standards as criteria of adequacy; (2) "hanging judge" patterns characterized by excessively vindictive, hateful, and unjust self-punitive reactions; and (3) eternal penance scenarios wherein persons endlessly resurrect old wrongdoings, punish themselves anew for them, and never forgive themselves.

PERFECTIONISM

It's the measuring stick that destroys.
PETER G. OSSORIO, personal communication, 1993

Jack, a rather articulate and introspective tax accountant, describes a self-critical scenario that he enacts almost daily: "On those rare occasions when a finished return looks good to me, I focus on how it wasn't done on time. If it was done on time, I focus on how inefficient I was in preparing it and how I've wasted money for my client and for my firm. If all that is okay, I focus on how I should have found a better way to do it. I always find something wrong. My standard is perfection, and if I achieve it, I get a '10.' If I fail to achieve it, I get a '0.' There are no 9.8s here like there are in Olympic figure skating."

It is customary in the clinical literature to regard the employment of a standard of perfection as, *ipso facto*, a self-destructive
practice (e.g., Burns, 1980; Hamachek, 1978; Rubin, 1975; Sorotzkin,
1985). The logical antidote to this practice then becomes helping individuals to abandon this standard and to adopt less stringent alternatives. Hamachek (1978), for example, advocates to his clients that
they "set reasonable, reachable goals for yourself," and "give yourself permission to be less than perfect" (p. 33). Utilizing this approach, some people may be weaned from perfectionistic standards
to their considerable benefit.

In the author's experience, however, the majority of perfectionistic individuals are loath to relinquish their standards. The modal
reason for this reluctance is that they regard such relinquishment as
an abandonment of their personal value for excellence and an unacceptable "settling" for mediocrity. Anyone who would ask them to
do so is asking them to compromise themselves. Such a client
stance places therapists in a difficult position. If they wish to urge a
relaxation of standards as described above, they are promoting a
therapeutic goal that runs strongly counter to the client's values
and desires, and they are thereby inviting resistance. With this practical difficulty in mind, a different perspective on the standard of
perfection will be adopted here, and one that generates considerably less resistance in most clients (see Chapter 8 for further discussion of the treatment issues involved here).

Many years ago, the theologian Reinhold Niebuhr raised the
question of the intent of the biblical injunction, "Be ye perfect!"
(Niebuhr, 1956). Was perfection intended, he inquired, to be something that people could actually achieve and were expected to
achieve? If so, the standard was quite impossible and therefore foolish. However, he suggested, perfection was being posed, not as a
standard of adequacy, but as an ideal—as a destination toward
which persons should strive even though it was understood that
they could never reach it. Like a guide star to an ancient navigator,
it would provide a constant direction for one's efforts but not an expectation of arrival. Failure to achieve this ideal would be inevitable, and the appropriate reaction in the face of such failure
would be, not self-condemnation and repudiation, but humility and
a renewed commitment to strive toward perfection.

The contrast between this perspective and the one contained in
my client's quote is stark. For Jack, perfection is not an ideal. It is a
standard of personal adequacy. Failure to achieve it is not occasion

for humble acknowledgment and renewed efforts. It is occasion to "give oneself a zero" and declare oneself a complete failure. One should achieve perfection (the note of grandiosity is unmistakable here), and failure to do so is grounds for recriminations against oneself (including, quite possibly, the sorts of self-degradations discussed in the previous chapter).

In the author's experience, it is not the pursuit of perfection per se that is a problem. Rather, it is its employment as a standard of adequacy, and often in every sphere of the individual's life (Hamachek, 1978), that proves so destructive. Where persons have a perspective in which it is understood that perfection is an unreachable ideal whose function is to give direction to their efforts, and that such an ideal should be employed in only a few select areas of life, they find this a viable arrangement.

There are four other common clinical scenarios that may be seen as variations on the perfectionistic theme. All of them entail employment of some standard of adequacy that, like perfection, dooms the person to failure all or most of the time. All share the identical formula that, "If I do not meet standard X, then I am a failure (defective, inadequate, unworthy, etc.)."

Standard: Being Number One

In this self-critical pattern, the individual's operative motto is: "Be number one, or you're nothing." The critic's stance is that it is imperative that one be the very best in some arena of life and perhaps in many or even all. If that arena is athletics, then one must be the champion. If it is school or work, then one must be the most brilliant or the most achieving. If it is social, one must be the best looking, have the best figure or physique, have the best personality, or be the most popular.

An example of the use of this standard is Michael, a successful graphic artist in his middle thirties. Among other presenting concerns, Michael reported a recurrent pattern that occurred whenever he attended parties or other social gatherings. Again and again on such occasions he would single out another male who had some outstanding characteristic. Perhaps the man would be quite handsome, or a gifted athlete, or a charming conversationalist, or the owner of a successful business. Whatever the man's singular gift or accomplishment, Michael would focus on it and would note how he himself was inferior to the man in this respect. He would then become very preoccupied with thoughts about how serious his own deficiency was and how he had better start working on that aspect of his life. The end result of this scenario was always the same. Michael would leave at the end of the evening feeling quite depressed, inferior, and deficient.

In this pattern, comparison with other people takes center stage, and any recognition that one fails the comparison is grounds for feeling deficient and inferior (McKay & Fanning, 1992; Rubin, 1975). Life becomes a series of contests where again there are only winners and losers—"tens and zeros but no 9.8s." The critic cannot make appraisals such as, "She's prettier than I am, but I feel okay about my looks," or "Being a captivating conversationalist like Joe isn't a strong point of mine, and I can live with that." Much less is the individual able simply to drop out of the whole game of comparison.

STANDARD: BEING GOD

The second variation on the perfectionistic theme has as its standard being a deity (Bergner, 1981; Rubin, 1975). The critic judges, in effect, that "If you have failed to be omnipotent and omniscient, you are a failure." Individuals do not of course run about saying such things as, "I expect myself to be God," or "If I am not all-knowing and all-powerful, then I am a failure." Rather, what is observable are self-criticisms that make sense as criticisms only when one realizes that the standards implicitly being upheld are omniscience or omnipotence. For example, an individual might condemn himself for making an error in a situation where, given the information available to him, such a mistake was unavoidable. The implicit claim in such a case is an omniscient one: "No matter that I could not have known; I should have known." Another individual might attack herself as somehow responsible for problematic behavior on the part of her child or spouse in a situation where such behavior is clearly beyond the province of her personal autonomy. The implicit claim here is an omnipotent one: "I can control the behavior of other persons." A third individual might castigate himself for a decision that, while undertaken carefully and prudently, did not turn out well. "I should have known" is the classic self-indictment here, and the standard upheld is prescience: "I should have been able to predict the future and thus to make a decision that would have proven more successful."

Standard: A Better Way

The third variation on the theme of unattainable standard setting might be termed "carrot dangling." The critic's formula here is "There is surely a better way to do what you did, and because you did not do it that way, you are a failure." Like the carriage driver of yore who dangled a carrot always a bit ahead of his mule, the critic here continually places the criterion of acceptability somewhere beyond what he or she in fact achieved. The individual in this scenario takes what amounts to a fact about the world—namely, that there will almost always be a better way to do something—and uses this fact as a way to disqualify what in fact was done or is the case. It is as if a computer designer, in the face of the fact that computer design is continually advancing, would never stop and appraise any new product as an excellent computer. Rather, what he or she would always conclude is that, "This is not a good computer because a better one is possible and some day will be built." The operating premise of critics who engage in this carrot-dangling pattern typically seems to be: "If I let myself be satisfied with anything I do, I will lapse into complacency; I must always dangle the standard of success higher to keep myself motivated."

Standard: Ceaseless Productivity

Daniel, an architect in his forties, relates the following: "It just seems like I have to be doing something 'productive' or 'constructive' all the time. If I try to do something like just sit and watch a football game or anything else that has no work value, I get depressed. If I try to read a book that's just a 'page turner' and has no educational value, same thing. It's like there's some little voice inside me telling me I'd better improve myself every single minute of the day, or I'd better do something 'worthwhile,' or else I'm being lazy and irresponsible and wasting my time."

This fourth and final variation on the perfectionist theme is one in which the critic upholds as a standard of adequacy that the person be ceaselessly engaged in activities with utilitarian value (Bergner, 1981; White, 1988). He or she must always be engaged in actions that are "constructive" or "educational" or "productive." What is ruled out in this scenario are inactivity and play. If the movie or book or television show does not better the person, if the game or other recreational pastime "doesn't accomplish anything," then engagement in it will be grounds for the individual to indict himself or herself as, in Daniel's words, "lazy and irresponsible and wasting my time." Such indictments will be meted out by many persons even at the end of a day where they have pushed themselves relentlessly and accomplished a great deal. As one young woman expressed the matter, "Even if I'm exhausted, if there are still things on my things-to-do list, I just can't relax and let them go until the next day."

Summary

The entire description of perfectionistic self-critical patterns may be summarized by turning the whole matter on its head and describing what it is that perfectionistic persons cannot do. They cannot let themselves be ordinary people (cf, Hamachek, 1978; Rubin, 1975). Such ordinary people, realizing that they have finite time and energy, decide on the basis of their value priorities where excellence (and even perfection) is to be pursued and where it is not. Further, they regard such perfection as something that they will rarely if ever achieve, but which nonetheless provides a direction for their best efforts. Finally, they recognize and accept that their lives inevitably will include failures, rejections, mistakes, personal weaknesses, deficient abilities, socially unacceptable feelings, and many more "imperfections;" and that these are merely part of the human condition, not grounds for declaring themselves abject, worthless, failures.

TYPICAL CONSEQUENCES OF PERFECTIONISM

This section presents a number of commonly observed consequences that are specific to perfectionistic patterns of standard setting. It should be noted, however, that these perfectionistic patterns often occur in conjunction with private self-degradation ceremonies ("I didn't do it perfectly; therefore, I'm stupid and inadequate"), and that they share some consequences with self-degradation even when the two patterns do not occur together. For these two reasons, consequences of perfectionistic self-critical acts overlap with those described in the previous chapter on self-degradation. These common consequences include feelings of personal ineligibility, behavioral restriction, and failure to generate any usable problem diagnoses and prescriptions for needed change. Because these consequences have already been discussed in Chapter 2, they will not be discussed again here.

Constant Failure

The first and most obvious consequence of employing perfection as a standard of adequacy is that it dooms individuals to almost constant failure (Hamachek, 1978; McKay & Fanning, 1992). Success is impossible or at best a rare occurrence, and so persons are forever "getting a zero" from themselves. Virtually nothing they do results in a sense that they have succeeded or in the feelings of pride, appreciation, or accomplishment that might accompany such a sense.

Demotivation

It should be clear from the previous point that there is very little self-reinforcement or self-acknowledgment in this perfectionistic scenario (Hamachek, 1978). Individuals essentially create for themselves a situation that is antithetical to personal motivation: "Why do anything when nothing is ever good enough?"

Disillusionment

To employ some standard X as a standard of personal adequacy is to take a certain stance vis-à-vis oneself: "I expect and insist on performance that meets standard X, and I will prosecute if I do not meet that standard." To expect, insist on, and hold myself responsible for meeting a standard of perfection is, when one thinks about it, to make a rather exalted claim; namely, that I am somebody who can attain such a standard. Thus, persons who hold themselves to perfectionistic standards are claiming in effect that they are persons who are capable of flawless performance, always being number one, being omniscient and omnipotent, always doing things in the absolute best way they could be done, and/or being ceaselessly productive. In what is often a subtle way, they are suffering from what might be termed "delusions of grandeur." "Deep down," some of the more articulate and insightful of them will say, "I really believe that I am this very specially and uniquely gifted individual who is not like other, ordinary people" (Rubin, 1975; Sorotzkin, 1985).

Seen from this vantage point, any given failure for the person is not merely a failure to meet some abstract standard of perfection. Rather, to recognize such a failure is to experience a painful comedown, a blow to one's pride (Kohut, 1971; Rubin, 1975; Sorotzkin, 1985). The message that the failure carries is that, "I'm not that special kind of person that I thought I was and that I feel I must be if I am to be worthwhile. I'm not beyond being rejected by others, or making foolish mistakes, or being bested by more gifted or intelligent people, or failing at something. And if I am not that, then, by my standards, I am nothing." The failure to be perfect then becomes grounds for very painful disillusionment and intense feelings of deficiency and inferiority.

FAILURE TO ACHIEVE THE SAFETY OF
BEING BEYOND REPROACH

A possible definition of the word "perfect" is "beyond criticism or reproach." If X is perfect, then there are no grounds for criticizing it, for finding it wanting. This linguistic consideration captures nicely an important psychological perspective of many perfectionistic persons. They impose their perfectionistic standards and are highly invested in their fulfillment, in part because it is so vitally important to them to place themselves beyond the dreaded reproaches of others (Ferrari, 1992; Sorotzkin, 1985; Stone & Stone, 1993; White, 1988). If they are perfect, then they succeed in achieving a position of safety, a position where no one can find them wanting. When they are imperfect, in contrast, they feel extremely vulnerable, endangered, and hyperconcerned that others will attack and devastate them.

For example, Mary, a highly perfectionistic social service worker in her late thirties, reported that she had forgotten a chore that she had agreed to do for her church and had been reminded by her pastor of her oversight. The chore was not a highly significant matter and occurred in a larger context in which she was an exceptionally active and giving parishioner. However, Mary became extremely distraught and preoccupied with this minor lapse because it left her feeling highly exposed to the criticism of others. Others, she was sure, would conclude from her mistake that she was "incompetent, unfit, and irresponsible." In the course of discussing this incident, Mary discerned that an extremely important reason why she held herself to perfectionistic standards was that she felt she had to make herself acceptable to other persons, and she felt so exposed, endangered, and humiliated whenever she believed that she had failed to do so.

Loss of Satisfactions Inherent in Participation

In perfectionistic scenarios, what tends to assume overwhelming importance for persons is the outcome of their efforts. Was the work or performance executed to perfection and did it place one beyond reproach? Was the A+ grade achieved? Did one win the contest/secure the highest rating/triumph over all the others for brilliance (attractiveness, charisma, sensitivity, etc.)? Relative to ordinary persons, the achievement of these outcomes assumes an inordinate and central importance. Failure to achieve them must be avoided at all costs. The infamous athletic slogan that "Winning isn't the most important thing—it's the only thing," captures this perspective nicely.

In contrast, what are conspicuous by their absence in perfectionistic scenarios are ongoing appreciations and satisfactions that derive from the *process* of participating in social practices (Rubin, 1975). To paraphrase the old saying, "getting there" is not only not "half the fun" for perfectionistic individuals, it is often no fun at all. As the considerations already mentioned attest, there is so much riding on the outcome, so much at stake, that it assumes an importance for the person that precludes relaxing and enjoying the ongoing process of participation. When winning is a life-and-death matter, it becomes extremely difficult to relax and enjoy the game.

Negative Focus

Perfectionistic patterns lend themselves to a negative attentional focus. What tends to draw the critic's attention are deficits from the standard upheld, not positive actions, accomplishments, or personal qualities that might be appreciated or even celebrated (Bergner, 1981; McKay & Fanning, 1992). For example, Daniel, the architect quoted previously who felt compelled to be ceaselessly productive, reported that no matter how much he might have accomplished on a given day, he would give scarcely any thought at all to it. The status of such accomplishments was that they were "behind him," mere "cross-offs on his things-to-do list." As a critic, his attitude toward himself was essentially, "What have you done for me lately?" At the end of each day, what captured his attention were the things that he had not gotten around to doing. Particularly if these were things that he had been avoiding, he related, he would be rather punitive with himself at the end of what might have been a highly productive day.

In these self-critical scenarios, individuals often seem to change the subject (of conversation or attention) in an almost reflexive fashion when there is the possibility of considering anything positive about themselves. This propensity can be seen in the quote from Jack at the beginning of this chapter. If he noted, however fleetingly, that a tax return had been prepared in a skillful way, he would immediately turn his attention to how it had not been done quickly enough or to some other negative factor. Other clients, when asked to consider their strengths or accomplishments, have responded that, "Well, yes, I suppose I did handle the interview well, but I upstaged my partner in doing so and that's all that I could think about afterward," and "Sure, I've built up a successful business; but what does that matter when I'm incapable of having a lasting, intimate relationship?"

DIMINISHED ACHIEVEMENT

Ironically, despite the fixation on extraordinary accomplishment in perfectionistic scenarios, there is much in them that is antithetical to such accomplishment. By way of analogy, one might consider the consequences of working under a boss who set impossible standards, was never satisfied with actual outcomes, noticed only problems and deficiencies, and routinely branded his employees abject failures. There is little reinforcement in such a scenario, and so an important incentive to achievement is missing. Second, such a management regime would lead many employees to become anxiously preoccupied with avoiding imperfect performances, which would frequently result in needless inefficiency, diminished productivity, and procrastination (Burns, 1980; Ferrari, 1992; Hamachek, 1978; White, 1988). Third, such a regime would for many workers lead in time to such responses as demoralization and burnout on the one hand or active rebellion on the other. The worker, striving strenuously for a success that never comes and taking no joy in the process of work itself, begins to experience the characteristic reaction of the burned-out individual: "I can't go on." Or, he or she begins to experience another characteristic response to tyrannical masters, that of rebellion against their dictates (Bergner, 1981).

EMOTIONAL CONSEQUENCES

The patterns that have been discussed in this section entail the setting of impossible standards, the use of an all-or-nothing "grading scale" such that the individual fails continually, an exclusive preoccupation with outcome at the expense of appreciating ongoing participation in life activities, and an attentional focus on lapses from perfection. It should not be surprising that the emotional consequences of such a way of life center primarily around depression, meaninglessness, and demoralization (Beck, 1976; Burns & Beck, 1978).

THE "HANGING JUDGE"

Randy, a 22-year-old journalism student, missed his highway turnoff one day on the way to school. The mistake was not a costly one, since the next turnoff, an alternative route to his destination, was only a mile down the road and he was under no time pressure. On recognizing his mistake, however, he had what he later described as a "fit" in which he screamed a long stream of obscenities at himself. So extreme was his self-directed anger that he shook his steering wheel violently and pounded his fist repeatedly on his dashboard.

Jack, the tax accountant mentioned previously, despised his job but felt trapped in it because he could see no alternative means by which he could maintain his excellent standard of living. All external indications such as annual evaluations, raises, and promotions indicated that, despite his disaffection, he did high-quality, conscientious work. In the context of an empty-chair exercise during one session, Jack was asked to adopt a critic stance and verbalize his evaluations of himself. In the role of critic, he angrily and contemptuously offered the following appraisal of himself as a worker: "He has no ambition—never puts in the extra effort. He never studies or reads a damned thing to improve himself. He doesn't concentrate at work. There's nothing he's really good at. His work is never any good. He's not worth the effort to waste my contempt on. He's lazy—like a welfare client after a free handout. I have no interest in helping him until he shows me something."

Originated by Ossorio (1976) (see also Driscoll, 1981, 1989), the image of the "hanging judge" is that of the old Western frontier judge who, for any offense regardless of how minor, would sentence the defendant to death by hanging. It is the image of someone bent not on seeking justice and seeing to it that the punishment fits the crime but on accomplishing the angry and vindictive destruction of the accused. Let us examine each of the three characteristics that, taken collectively, comprise the hanging judge syndrome: self-hatred, injustice, and lack of compassion for oneself.

SELF-HATRED

What distinguishes the hanging judge form of self-criticism (which again may occur empirically in isolation or in conjunction with other patterns) is its overly harsh, vindictive, prosecutorial quality. What is observed here is not the quiet, sinking-sensation quality that may characterize, for example, some persons as they draw negative comparisons between themselves and others. Rather, what is evident are qualities of hatred, rage, and assaultiveness of persons toward themselves, qualities that have led previous authors to describe these persons as "abusive" critics and even as "killer" critics (Stone & Stone, 1993, p. 85; see also Rubin, 1975).

INJUSTICE

The self-critical attacks at issue here seem to the dispassionate observer to be seriously out of proportion to the significance of the alleged offense. The response of Randy described above typifies this draconian quality. For something as factually inconsequential as a missed highway turnoff that caused him a five-minute delay, Randy launched an enraged, hateful diatribe against himself that was replete with all manner of self-degradation and obscene name-calling.

LACK OF COMPASSION FOR SELF

Finally, as the example of Jack illustrates, there is little interest in this scenario in helping oneself, only interest in punishing and reviling oneself (Driscoll, 1981; Ossorio, 1976; Stone & Stone, 1993). In persons who exhibit other patterns of destructive self-criticism, one will frequently hear a note struck of "I criticize myself this way because I believe that it benefits me." Although the person might be mistaken in his or her calculations of what is helpful, still there is an intent to act in one's own best interest that lies behind the criticism. In hanging judge patterns, evidence of such self-beneficial intentions are notably absent. The spirit in which the criticism is rendered seems more one of "I hate and am furious with myself and wish to punish myself severely by venting my anger and my hatred." The hanging judge, to return to the metaphor, is a judge whose attitude toward those convicted is: "I don't give a damn about rehabilitating them; I just want them to pay in spades for what they've done."

CONSEQUENCES

Persons who engage heavily in this hanging judge pattern of self-criticism usually encounter two primary consequences. The first of these is depression. In the wake of their angry, abusive attacks upon themselves, such individuals characteristically report being seriously depressed and, in extreme cases, suicidal (Stone & Stone, 1993). Such consequences are consistent with the classical psychoanalytic contention that depression is caused by anger directed against one's own person (Fenichel, 1945; Freud, 1917/1958; Rado, 1929; Rubin, 1975). The second consequence is a notable absence of corrective action. Again, as in the case of private self-degradation, there is no corrective element (and, as noted above, no corrective motivation) in this self-critical scenario. Typical self-critical attacks, as exemplified by those of Randy and Jack, contain no useful problem diagnoses or prescriptions for how to remedy what has gone wrong. Overall, then, in the aftermath of a critic attack, the individual is left feeling quite depressed, personally savaged, and possessed of few ideas or motivations pertaining to the remediation of his or her alleged mistakes and failings.

ETERNAL PENANCE

The playwright Tennessee Williams once stated in a televised interview that he had been deeply troubled all of his life by something that he had done as a teenager. On his younger sister's birthday, he had said something very cruel and spiteful to her, caused her to cry, and ruined her birthday. Decades later, at the time of the interview, he related that he had recalled this incident countless times over the years, had experienced a fresh and very painful sense of remorse each time, and had never forgiven himself for what he had done.

Like Tennessee Williams, some clients become mired in a pattern of endless self-recrimination for their wrongdoings. They continually resurrect past misdeeds, criticize themselves anew for them, and experience again the guilt, shame, humiliation, or other emotion that has always accompanied these recollections (Driscoll, 1981; McKay & Fanning, 1992; Rubin, 1975). For these persons, there is no self-forgiveness and therefore no putting the matter to rest. They are like judges in the legal system who would try a defendant, find her guilty, and punish her—and then retry, reconvict, and repunish her again and again for the same crime.

In our culture, as in most (Ossorio & Sternberg, 1981), there is a social practice of atonement. While this practice is paradigmatically interpersonal, its description is quite helpful in grasping precisely what is involved in eternal penance scenarios. The situation that calls for the social practice of atonement to be enacted is one in which an individual violates a community standard, and thus provides the community with reason to lower her standing with them or even, in extreme cases, to exclude her (Camden, 1993; Ossorio & Sternberg, 1981; cf. Snyder & Higgins, 1988). A clinically familiar example of such a situation is one where the community in question is a married couple, and the violation is an infidelity that has caused the betrayed partner to leave the relationship and to contemplate divorce. A second example would be one in which the community in question is a religious one, the violation a serious sin against that community's moral precepts, and the reaction one of ostracizing (excommunicating) the offender.

In this situation, the transgressor may attempt to atone for the wrongdoing. That is, he or she may attempt to do what is necessary to try to regain his or her pretransgression standing in the community (Camden, 1993; Ossorio & Sternberg, 1981). Transgressors may attempt to gain such reconciliation or reinstatement by such actions as (1) openly acknowledging their wrongdoing, (2) expressing sorrow, regret, and remorse for what they have done (i.e., apologizing), and (3) declaring their intent never to repeat the action. Further, since actions are generally taken to be more valid indicators of a person's sincerity than mere words, they may (4) voluntarily undertake some sort of penance (i.e., some punishment or hardship) as a further and stronger expression of their remorse and intent to change, and/or (5) make voluntary restitution for their wrongdoing where this is possible (Ossorio & Sternberg, 1981).

In the face of such penitential behavior by the transgressor, the community has an absolutely essential role to play if the social practice of atonement is to come to a successful completion. That role is to scrutinize the transgressor's behavior and, if they are satisfied, to declare to him or her: "We recognize from your words and actions that indeed you do subscribe to our standards, that you do regret your violation, and do intend in future to commit yourself to our standards. You are forgiven and are regarded once again as one of us, as a member in good standing of our community. Go in peace: the matter is at an end" (see Baron, 1990; Ohbuchi, Kameda, & Agarie, 1989, on the effects of apologies on offended parties).

From the foregoing, it is clear that this entire ceremony of forgiveness and reinstatement to full standing cannot come to completion without the final community affirmation. It may be noted further that this affirmation rests on a critic act—on an appraisal that indeed the individual does subscribe to important standards, does intend to do better, has shown good faith by making sufficient amends, and so forth. Alternatively, there are times when this appraisal takes into account the presence of mitigating factors (e.g., the presence of accident, extraordinary circumstance, or atypical states) that seem pertinent to an assessment of the transgressor's standing (cf. Snyder et al., 1983).

In eternal penance scenarios, one person is both the aggrieved other and the transgressor—the accuser and the accused. In these scenarios, individuals as accusers have been unwilling or unable to forgive themselves as transgressors. An illuminating and therapeutically useful way to redescribe eternal penance scenarios is to say that in them individuals have been unable to make, on their own behalf, the sorts of restorative critic appraisals described above. They have been unable to look at themselves and to conclude that they do subscribe to the transgressed standard in their behavior, are genuinely regretful for their violation, have made sufficient amends in forms such as restitution or penance, and/or were subject to the influence of mitigating factors. Whatever the reason (and these may include the actual absence of some of these requisite elements), these persons have never been able to look at themselves and to reappraise themselves as worthy of reinstatement to full moral standing in the human community. Thus, they have not been able to bring these penitential matters to completion and say to themselves in effect: "Be at peace; the matter is at an end."

CONCLUSION

To this point, the focus of this book has been primarily on descriptive matters. Four patterns of pathological self-criticism and their destructive consequences for persons have been described. These have included (1) private self-degradation ceremonies, (2) the employment of various perfectionistic standards as criteria of personal adequacy, (3) engagement in "hanging judge" behaviors marked by excessively hateful and unjust attacks on self, and (4) the endless resurrection of old "crimes" for which individuals cannot forgive themselves. In the experience of the author, and in the clinical literature, these four patterns emerge as the most common forms that pathological self-criticism assumes.

The focus of this book will now shift from descriptive to explanatory and procedural matters. In the next chapter, the core question that will be addressed is this: If clients are destructively criticizing themselves in the ways described heretofore, how may we best assess both what they are doing and why they are doing it?

CHAPTER 4

ASSESSING SELF-CRITICAL PATTERNS AND THE FACTORS MAINTAINING THEM

RAYMOND M. BERGNER AND
CYNTHIA A. GOOD MOJAB

Pragmatics stands as the essential criterion, for the principle standard for adequate assessment is that it contain what is required for the [therapeutic] tasks at hand.

RICHARD DRISCOLL (1984, p. 126)

The focus of this chapter is the assessment of all of those factors that, in a given case, are pertinent to selecting effective strategies of intervention. Once general inquiry has revealed that pathological self-criticism is at the heart of a client's problems and is to be the focus of therapeutic efforts, two general areas must be assessed. The first of these is the precise nature of the patterns of self-criticism being exhibited by the individual. Is he or she engaging in self-degradation, the imposition of perfectionistic standards, excessive harshness and punitiveness, eternally penitential behavior, or some other idiosyncratic pattern? The second area for assessment is factors that influence the individual to do what he or she is doing. This category includes (1) the purposes or goals that individuals are trying to achieve by their pathological self-critical behavior, (2) the specific situations that tend to elicit this behavior, (3) pertinent elements from their social learning histories, and (4) influences from the broader culture.

While the focus in this chapter will be on assessment, it should be noted that many of the procedures described also qualify as interventions. When therapist and client collaborate in these procedures, both of them glean useful information. For the client, both the possession of this information and many of the processes by which it is obtained frequently result in behavioral change. Assessment here is very much interwoven with intervention (Driscoll, 1984).

ASSESSING SELF-DIRECTED CRITIC ACTS AND HELPING INDIVIDUALS TO RECOGNIZE THEM

In order to change their pathological modes of criticizing themselves, persons must first recognize them (Driscoll, 1984; McKay & Fanning, 1992; Stone & Stone, 1993). They must observe precisely what they are doing to themselves in this respect. They cannot change what they cannot observe or recognize. At the outset of therapy, there are significant differences in how well different clients are able to identify their destructive self-critical patterns of behavior. At one extreme are persons who are quite self-observant in this regard. All of the individuals who were quoted in previous chapters—e.g., Jack, who reported on his "10 or 0" scale; Randy, who described his fit of rage in his car; and Shannon, who related her self-assigned "slut" label and its implications—were good observers and articulate describers of their own self-critical practices. With such individuals, it is generally a relatively easy matter to tease out, for our assessment purposes and for theirs, a precise picture of how they function as critics of themselves.

At the other end of the continuum are persons who are relatively unable to observe themselves as critics (Driscoll, 1981). Their reports about themselves may assume forms such as the following: "Sometimes, for reasons I can't put my finger on, I just get this horrible sinking feeling that I am so unimportant to others." "When I am around her, I don't know why, but I always come away feeling so awful and so inferior." "My father made what seemed like a minor critical remark, but somehow it just sent me spiraling down into depression." The general picture in these cases is that individuals are able to report the consequences of their self-critical acts—the depression, low self-esteem, vulnerability to criticism, and so forth—but not the acts themselves. The sense created in them is that their pain emanates from unknown sources, or that it "comes from out of nowhere."

The latter individuals are in a very poor position from which to change. They have a serious problem but they are unacquainted with what might be termed its "business end" (Bergner, 1993). They know the effects, but not the cause of these effects. Are these causes medical? marital? something deep-seated from their childhood? Unlike the cartoon character Pogo, who once stated that "We have met the enemy and he is us" (Kelly, 1981, p. 203), they do not know their "enemies," and thus they have no conception regarding where they might best launch an effective "counterattack." Therefore, the therapist must help them to recognize both the fact that they are the perpetrators of their own misery and the precise details regarding the nature of their self-critical acts.

There are a number of factors to consider when attempting to assess the destructive self-critical practices of persons who cannot readily identify them and to help these persons to recognize what they are doing to themselves. In the following section, these factors are examined and a variety of assessment tactics designed to address them are presented.

INSTANTANEOUS, AUTOMATIC APPRAISALS

Human beings are capable of instantaneous, automatic appraisals, and in fact make them constantly and routinely (Uleman & Bargh, 1989). For example, when speaking, a person might appraise that the word "well," rather than the word "good," is called for in a sentence. Typically, this person will just say "well" in the course of uttering the sentence and be unaware of having made the discrimination, much less of any self-statements to the effect that "This sentence calls for an adverb, not an adjective." It is the same for countless human appraisals (e.g., for virtually every word in every spoken sentence, and for most of our minute-to-minute decisions as automobile drivers to stop, shift, or accelerate). They are made instantaneously, automatically, and with little or no awareness.

Very often, critic acts take the form of such instantaneous and automatic appraisals. Their authors quickly, automatically, and with negligible awareness make critical evaluations of themselves (cf. Beck et al., 1979; Beck & Emery, 1985; Haaga & Beck, 1992, on "automatic thoughts"). Here, there will be no self-statements to be found along the lines of "My quietness at this party is further evidence that I am a complete social incompetent with nothing of interest to say to others." Rather, the only clues to be found that such a verdict has been rendered may be the feelings of depression, inferiority, and personal insufficiency experienced by the person during and after the party. Thus, when instantaneous destructive self-appraisals have been made, it will be very difficult for their authors to observe and recognize their precise nature and, consequently, to report this in psychotherapy.

Assessment Procedure: Logical Reconstruction

Where destructive critic acts consist of such instantaneous appraisals, one assessment tactic that may be employed profitably is that of logical reconstruction. Just as one might reason that, "From the way you constructed your sentence, you must have judged that an adverb was called for," so a therapist might reason that, "From the withdrawal, depression, and despair you are describing, it sounds like you judged that you were inferior to her and that there could be no possibility of her being interested in you." Such critical appraisals may be hypothesized and discussed with the client, and in this way their likely content and nature may be determined. The work here is analogous to that of a detective who must start with the facts of the accomplished crime and then work backward to reconstruct what must have happened (cf. Beck & Weishaar, 1989, on employing *post hoc* deduction to infer schemas from automatic thoughts). When such collaborative work with clients bears fruit, they can become aware of the nature and content of their self-critical acts, can see how they are their perpetrators, and can take an essential first step toward removing them from their instantaneous, "automatic pilot" mode of perpetration (Bergner, 1993).

DEFICIENT OBSERVER FUNCTION

Many persons are poor observers of themselves (Driscoll, 1981; Ossorio, 1976). They are not very able to take an observational stance in relation to their own thinking (and often to their behavior in general) and to see clearly what they are doing. Unable to observe their own self-critical acts, they repeatedly find themselves with unanswered question such as the following: "Why do I feel so bad every time I visit my friend Martha?" "Why do I sometimes get depressed when nothing bad seems to have happened?" "Why do the criticisms of others seem to devastate me so much?" For these persons, the answers to such questions could be determined were they better able to observe themselves.

Assessment Procedure: Self-Monitoring

An excellent technique, both for assessing self-critical behavior and for helping persons to become better observers of themselves, is that of self-monitoring (Ciminero, Nelson, & Lipinski, 1977; Haaga & Beck, 1992; Rehm & Rokke, 1988). Widely and successfully used by cognitive and behavioral therapists, the details of this procedure vary somewhat depending on the theoretical orientation of the therapist and the situation with which he or she is confronted. However, the basic technique generally involves instructing clients to observe carefully their own therapeutically relevant behavior or emotions, to note their association with other states of affairs such as preceding and ensuing events, and to record these observations for discussion in subsequent therapeutic sessions.

In the author's work with self-critical individuals, self-monitoring usually assumes the following form. It is suggested to clients that they carry around a small index card. At those times when they realize that they are feeling emotionally upset or engaging in problematic behavior (e.g., withdrawing or lashing out angrily), they are to try to discern the nature of (1) their troublesome emotions or behaviors, (2) the events preceding these, and (3) their own thinking processes immediately prior to their problematic reactions. If they can identify these, they are to record their observations briefly on the index card. These notes are then brought to the following therapeutic session for discussion of their contents. From them, important themes regarding both the form and the content of the individual's specific patterns of destructive self-criticism may be discerned.

Aside from its assessment functions, self-monitoring serves a number of other highly useful ones. First, persons who meet with some success in this activity become more cognizant of the fact that their problems do not come from "out of the blue." They see clearly that they are the perpetrators of these problems through their self-criticism, and that they are not the helpless victims of some inexplicable, mysterious malady over which they have no control. They see, in Pogo's terms, both that "the enemy is us" and the precise nature of his or her "attacks."

Second, it is widely recognized that the behavior of monitoring oneself will often result by itself in decreases in the frequency of the monitored behavior (Ciminero et al., 1977; Rehm & Rokke, 1988).

These "reactive effects" of self-monitoring seem particularly evident in cases where the target behavior is a disvalued one and the individual is strongly motivated to discontinue it (Ciminero et al., 1977; Rehm & Rokke, 1988). Such a situation is often one that exists when clients discover the precise nature of their destructive self-critical practices. When they discern what they are doing, and that it is so debilitating, this alone frequently results in some diminution of the behavior.

Third and finally, the practice of self-monitoring may be paired at a later point with active attempts to combat destructive self-critical acts. Here clients are directed, not merely to discern how they are functioning as critics on specific occasions, but to make strong efforts to cease doing so and to engage in more constructive alternative behaviors (Beck et al., 1979; Haaga & Beck, 1992; McKay & Fanning, 1992). This procedure will be discussed at greater length in Chapter 7.

Assessment Procedure: Interviewing the Critic

The technique of interviewing the critic is helpful both in cases where persons are not good observers of their own critic functioning and in cases where their appraisals are so instantaneous and automatic as to be undetectable. The procedure entails asking individuals to abandon the ordinary practice of being themselves in the therapy hour and speaking in the first person (e.g., "I've been pretty depressed this week"). Instead, they are asked to be their own critics in the hour and to speak of themselves in the third person (e.g., "All John [the person himself] ever thinks about is himself").

An example may be helpful here to convey the general nature of this technique. A young woman, Beth, was having a very difficult time responding to questions about what she was thinking one evening when she sat down to watch television and found herself becoming quite depressed. Because this line of inquiry was getting nowhere, a change of assessment strategies seemed indicated, and the following directive was given: "When I ask you what you were thinking about when you became so upset, you are drawing a blank. You're saying, 'I just don't know what I was thinking—I didn't seem to be thinking anything at all.' Well, let's see if we can come at this thing in a little different way. This may seem a little strange but let me ask you to give it a try, and if it's too uncomfortable we can stop. I'd like to kind of 'split you in two.' The two parts are basically Beth and Beth's critic. Now over in this chair, let's put one of you—okay, that's where Beth sits. Now over here you are

Beth's critic. Okay, from this critic chair, I want to know what you think of Beth. And let's go back to the other night, when around eight o'clock or so Beth started watching television even though all of her chores weren't done. Right now, think of her sitting there watching TV. What do you think of her and of what she's doing?"

The basic technique to get at the individual's self-critical behaviors, then, is not to try to reconstruct, remember, or monitor anything. It is simply to request that the client adopt the role of critic and do a critique of himself or herself. The interview may be carried on in this fashion for whatever period of time is required to meet therapeutic ends. Often (including in the case just mentioned), the individual's critic functioning can be ascertained in this way when other methods fail.

Finally, to shift briefly from assessment to treatment matters, it may be noted that, when one interviews clients in their critic roles, one removes them from low-power, perceived victim positions and relocates them to high-power, perpetrator ones (Bergner, 1981, 1993). Consider, for example, the difference between asking a client, "Are you still in the grips of that depression?" and asking him or her, "What is your assessment of how you performed in that situation?" The former question addresses the person as a more or less passive recipient or victim of something beyond his or her control. The latter question addresses itself to—indeed calls upon the person to be—the person who is perpetrating certain forms of self-mistreatment that are resulting in depression. The utilization of this perpetrator position for therapeutic gain will be explored in greater detail in Chapter 5.

ASSESSING OWNERSHIP OF CRITIC BEHAVIORS

Frequently, individuals will get to a point where they recognize the self-critical actions at the root of their problems. However, when conveying their understanding of this, they will use expressions such as "my critic" or "my critical parent part," as if the behavior in question issues from some dissociated entity within them but not really from them (Cramerus, 1990). In the same vein, they may say things like, "She (the critic) has been quiet lately and given me a reprieve, but I'm always afraid she'll come back." Not only do such statements convey that the critic is "not me," but they convey a complete lack of perceived control over critic behaviors. They convey a sense that "This isn't my behavior that I can elect to do or not do; it issues from some part of me that I do not control."

Such persons must be helped to own their critic acts. That is, they must come to a full recognition that they are their authors or perpetrators—the same sort of recognition that "I am doing this" that they ordinarily have when they engage in the vast majority of their intentional actions. Individuals who perceive these criticisms as somehow inflicted on them by agencies beyond their personal control remain in low-power positions from which change is very difficult. Those who appreciate fully that they are active, responsible perpetrators of critic acts occupy positions of greater control from which change is far more possible. Essentially, from the latter position, desisting from destructive criticism and initiating other more constructive sorts becomes an active possibility (Bergner, 1981, 1993).

For these reasons, it is vitally important to assess the degree of personal ownership of critic behaviors experienced by the individual. Should this sense prove deficient, the assessments discussed in the next section, as well as many techniques discussed in later chapters, are helpful in facilitating much fuller senses of personal authorship and control.

ASSESSING WHAT CLIENTS ARE TRYING TO ACCOMPLISH WITH SELF-CRITICISM

Criticizing oneself is a purposive act. It is engaged in by persons to achieve certain desired ends (Driscoll, 1981, 1989; McKay & Fanning, 1992; Stone & Stone, 1993). Further, an understanding of what clients are trying to accomplish with their self-critical behavior is central to the modification of this behavior. This section addresses many reasons why this is so, beginning with the importance of persons owning and taking control of their behavior.

When clients are reluctant to own their critical actions, they usually have important reasons not to recognize fully that it is they who are behaving this way. These reasons generally have to do with not wanting to recognize that they are acting in ways that seem stupid, malicious, and/or mentally disturbed. The most helpful therapeutic attitude to counter this resistance is one that conveys, "I assume that you must have some very good reasons for behaving as you do. You wouldn't do the things you are doing to yourself un-

less you thought that they would accomplish some important purposes." The self-critical behavior is reframed as a good faith attempt to accomplish worthwhile ends (Driscoll, 1981, 1989; McKay
& Fanning, 1992; Stone & Stone, 1993), and the therapist can then
proceed to inquire about these ends. Once clients appreciate their
positive reasons for criticizing themselves as they have, they are
generally far readier to recognize that it is they who behave this
way.

In addition to helping clients to own their self-critical actions,
knowing what they are trying to accomplish with those actions
achieves a number of other vital therapeutic benefits. First, once individuals are aware of what they are trying to achieve, they are in a
better position to evaluate their operating premises that "criticizing
myself this way will bring me benefits X, Y, and Z." For as long as
these operating premises remain unarticulated, they cannot be subjected to evaluation. Once the individual is aware of them, however,
certain questions may be raised: "Has treating myself this way in
fact secured for me these ends or has it not? Has it secured them but
at too high a personal cost in terms of emotional pain, low self-esteem, and restricted living?" When clients raise such questions,
they typically realize that their critical practices have not been particularly successful in getting them what they sought, or that these
practices have achieved limited success but at far too high a cost.

Second, once clients' existing motivations have been determined, the therapist may enlist them in the service of change.
Specifically, individuals may be shown how alternative critic behaviors might do a better job of getting them what they have been
seeking all along, and do so without the pain and destructiveness
inherent in their old practices. As Buckminster Fuller once advocated, "Don't oppose forces; use them" (1985, p. 153).

Third, when some clients recognize that their self-critical behaviors are rational ones designed to accomplish worthwhile purposes, they achieve a very reassuring realization that behaving and
feeling as they have does not mean that they are mentally ill. As
Raimy (1975) demonstrated in his excellent work on "phrenopho-
bia," the belief that one is mentally ill is enormously self-undermin-
ing. Furthermore, he observed, people are most likely to hold this
belief in circumstances where they are engaging in problematic behavior or experiencing extreme emotion without apparent sufficient reason. Thus, when clients who have been laboring under
such fears and beliefs can see that their behavior is engaged in for
reasons and that in fact it constitutes an effort to secure understand-

able and even laudable human ends, they simultaneously cease to believe that they are mentally ill.

The following sections address the more common purposes that clients are attempting to achieve with their self-critical behaviors. These purposes have been included based on the first author's clinical experience and the observations of other investigators (Driscoll, 1981, 1984, 1989; McKay & Fanning, 1992; Stone & Stone, 1993).

TO ACHIEVE SELF-IMPROVEMENT

Many clients believe that their favored modes of self-criticism will result in self-improvement, and that failure to implement them will result in complacency, stagnation, and repeated failure. If they do not denounce themselves for failure to meet the highest standards, vilify themselves for their mistakes, or bring home to themselves the "truth" about what degraded creatures they are, they believe that they will never achieve the improvements that in their minds they so desperately need (Driscoll, 1981, 1989; McKay & Fanning, 1992).

A commonly encountered form of this general self-improvement agenda is one where individuals believe that in order to avoid repeating past mistakes, they should make sure they never forget them. To accomplish this end, they continually remind themselves of them and berate themselves anew. Driscoll (1984, p. 219) uses an image he terms "wrong keys" to capture this agenda. In this image, he compares the self-critical individual with a pianist who attempts to improve her performance by keeping all of her previous mistakes in mind and reminding herself of just how bad they were. She focuses on remembering the "wrong keys" as her ticket to self-improvement. The image, which Driscoll uses with his clients, serves to clarify both the nature of the motivation and the fallacy inherent in it. To do something well, he notes, it is generally necessary to concentrate on doing it well and not to clutter one's mind and raise one's anxiety by thinking of all the possible ways that one might go wrong (cf. Frost & Henderson, 1991).

TO AVOID EGOTISM

Many persons believe that it is morally wrong to think well of themselves. In their view, to recognize a personal strength or accomplishment or to "pat themselves on the back" for anything is to be unacceptably egotistical, self-aggrandizing, conceited, or boastful. Many will say that they refrain from such public, and even private, behavior so as "not to get a big head." A few will say that they do not want to commit "the sin of pride."

In contrast, behaviors such as putting oneself down, refusing ever to be satisfied, downgrading one's strengths and accomplishments, and the like are seen by these persons as positively virtuous. To behave in such ways is to be humble, modest, unpretentious, or to "not take oneself too seriously." They cannot distinguish between these widely acknowledged virtues and destructive practices such as self-degradation and self-abuse. They cannot find the borderline between humility and self-mistreatment.

To Protect Themselves from Dangers

Often, clients sense that there are certain dangers that would ensue should they think more positively of themselves (Driscoll, 1981, 1989; McKay & Fanning, 1992; Stone & Stone, 1993). To avoid such dangers, they must take the "safe" path of engaging in destructive self-criticism. Among the more common dangers that persons report are the following.

Danger: Getting "Shot Down"

Some persons believe that if they raise themselves up, they run the risk of being "shot down" and humiliated (Driscoll, 1981, 1989; Godfrey, Jones, & Lord, 1986; McKay & Fanning, 1992). Were they, for example, to report personal successes or strengths to another, they might give the other reason to envy or resent them or to think them conceited and wish to "put them in their place." On the other hand, if they run themselves down to others by reporting their weaknesses and failures, they stake out a position of relative safety from attack (see Berglas & Jones, 1978; Higgins, Snyder, & Berglas, 1990, on the advantages of "self-handicapping behavior"). It is a commonly understood social obligation that one should never "beat a man when he's already down."

Danger: Having One's Hopes·Dashed

It can be a painful experience to be expecting something very good to happen and then to have one's hopes and expectations dashed when it is not forthcoming. Virtually all people can recall such painful instances from their childhoods and from other periods of their lives. Further, some will have adopted an explicit personal policy for averting this sort of letdown: "I don't ever let my-self get my hopes up; it is far better not to expect too much in life because then you can't be too disappointed."

A number of clients apply this general logic where self-criti-cism is concerned (Driscoll, 1981, 1989). Should they think well of themselves—should they see themselves, for example, as bright or capable or desirable to others—they would thereby be raising their hopes and expectations and dreams. But in the bargain, they be-lieve, they would be "setting themselves up" and exposing them-selves to the dangers of bitter hurt and disappointment. Far better, they conclude, to think little of oneself, expect little, and thus both avoid the pain of disappointment and even create the possibility of pleasant surprises.

Danger: Engaging in Hazardous Behavior

Grier and Cobbs (1968), in their study of African-American families prior to the black equality movement, observed that many mothers who were usually loving and nurturant would on occasion turn harshly critical and demeaning toward their male children. In explaining this seeming inconsistency, Grier and Cobbs hypothe-sized that the intent of this ostensibly destructive criticism was to teach the boys "their place" in society so as to promote their safety. Should the boys be allowed to see themselves as equal with whites, they might assert themselves in the face of discriminatory treatment and thereby run the risk of being badly beaten or even killed.

The logic of these mothers is the logic assumed by some per-sons who employ destructive self-criticism (Driscoll, 1981, 1989; McKay & Fanning, 1992). They believe that a good opinion of them-selves would create the danger that they would embark on some dangerous course of action. If they believed themselves attractive and desirable, they might imperil themselves by pursuing an extra-marital affair. If they regarded themselves as bright and competent, they might be tempted to leave the safety of their disliked yet se-cure jobs. If they appraised themselves as relatively blameless in some marital problem, they might endanger themselves by con-fronting their partner for the first time about his or her actions. Far better, such persons believe, to maintain control over themselves by a lowly estimate of their personal eligibilities and entitlements.

Danger: Criticism from Others

As noted in the previous chapter, many individuals privately criticize themselves in order to place themselves beyond the dreaded reproaches of others (Ferrari, 1992; Sorotzkin, 1985; Stone & Stone, 1993; White, 1988). For these individuals, an important purpose of self-criticism is to guide themselves to a position of safety where they have covered all the bases and not left themselves open to the danger of incurring the anger and criticisms of others. The critic's agenda is: "I must scrutinize myself, detect all possible grounds upon which others might find me wanting, dislike me, or reject me and get myself in line so that such dreaded things do not happen."

TO ATONE FOR PAST SINS

As noted in the previous chapter, the self-critical behavior of some persons assumes the form of reminding themselves again and again of their past transgressions and berating themselves anew (Driscoll, 1981, 1989; McKay & Fanning, 1992; Rubin, 1975). Consistent with that previous description, the primary purpose individuals seem bent on achieving with this behavior is to atone for these transgressions. In effect, they are doing again and again what penitents do: acknowledging and repudiating their wrongdoing, expressing their remorse, affirming that the transgressed standards do count with them, and undergoing self-inflicted punishment. Unfortunately, they are unable to provide the sorts of restorative critic appraisals that are needed to bring the process of atonement to completion, and thus to remove the need to repeat it.

TO MAINTAIN A NEEDED SENSE
OF SPECIALNESS AND SUPERIORITY

When one examines the self-critical acts of some clients, one discovers that they contain implicit claims to specialness and superiority (Ossorio, 1976; Rubin, 1975; Sorotzkin, 1985). Such claims are nicely illustrated in the apocryphal story of an ordinary citizen who, while sitting in his corner bar one evening watching the news, hears that war has broken out in the Middle East. Upon hearing this, he pounds his fist on the bar in anger and castigates himself in the following way: "I'm so mad at myself. If I had called the Secretary of State today, this wouldn't have happened" (from Ossorio, 1976, p. 129). On the surface, we see a man who is very angry and critical of himself. On closer inspection, we recognize the grandiosity of the claim this man is making to us: that a phone call from him could have altered the course of world events that day.

It is often the same with clients. When they castigate themselves for lapses from perfection, for example, they are often making the implicit claim that: "I am somebody for whom perfection is a possibility." When they lacerate themselves for the misbehavior or failure of others in certain contexts, they are making the implicit claim that "I am so powerful that I can control the behavior of others; I am like the mythical Atlas—I hold up the world."

There are also claims to specialness and superiority inherent in being a critic whose standards are so exalted and refined that all is found wanting. The drama critic sniffs and says, "Well, perhaps you found the play satisfactory; for myself I found it rather flawed." This delicious one-up move has its subtle parallels in the way some persons uphold their perfectionistic standards. For them, superior standards are the mark of superior persons, and to abjure such standards would render them ordinary and commonplace, a prospect that they find abhorrent and frightening (see Sorotzkin, 1985, on self-criticism in narcissistic individuals). Often, these persons will exhibit double standards for themselves and others. They hold themselves to elevated requirements, but hold others to ordinary ones. Again, claims to special person status may be detected here. As one client put the matter: "The standards that apply to ordinary people will not do—I adopt a higher standard for myself." Finally, from this position of superiority, clients may reject their own imperfect actions as somehow beneath them and thereby maintain a needed position of superiority even in the face of their flawed, finite human actions (Driscoll, 1981, 1989).

To Secure Reassurance and Sympathy

On a visit to a Hollywood studio a few years back, I had the opportunity to witness the work of one of the premier movie stars of the 1940s. This woman, now in her 60s, had been reduced to playing a supporting role in a much-maligned television adventure series, and it was a rehearsal for this show that I witnessed. At the end of each take, the former star would walk off the set berating herself aloud for how poorly she had performed her role in the scene. In response to this, other members of the cast would respond consistently by saying such things as, "Oh, no, you were absolutely wonderful," or "Nobody else could have done that scene the way you just did it; you're the real pro here."

Self-criticism is used by many persons as a means to secure reassurance and/or sympathy from others (Driscoll, 1981, 1989). Like the former movie queen, these individuals find that when they denigrate themselves to their spouses, friends, or family members, the latter (at least for a while) will tend to pay attention, to console them, and to say positive things about them. These self-critics, essentially unable to supply much in the way of affirmation or support for themselves, find that by externalizing their self-criticisms they can secure much-needed support and affirmation from other persons.

Powers and Zuroff (1988) conducted an empirical investigation of what tends to happen when individuals run themselves down to others. They found that experimental confederates who engaged in overt self-denigrating behavior frequently received public responses from others that were positive (e.g., higher ratings of their performance and positive conversational comments). However, they received private responses from others that were negative (e.g., they were perceived as poorly functioning individuals). Thus, those clients who engage in demeaning self-presentations to others may indeed frequently receive positive public outcomes, but they may pay a considerable hidden cost for this in terms of losing the high regard of others.

To Express Hostility

Some persons, especially ones who are restricted in their ability to do so more directly, may use self-criticism to express hostility. Driscoll (1984, p. 229) cites the example of a client of his who had spent several hours preparing a gourmet meal for her husband. The husband arrived home late, ate in silence, and commented only that the duck seemed a little dry. In response to this, his wife became extremely distraught, proclaimed loudly that she was a terrible cook who never did anything right, and ran sobbing from the table. Her self-criticism, however, contained an implicit hostile message to her husband: "See what your callousness and insensitivity have done to me; look how upset you've made me with myself." Further, this message was delivered in a way that was likely to disarm him and thus avoid a feared counterattack.

To Reduce the Demands and Expectations of Others

Some individuals criticize themselves because they fear that others will hold them responsible or expect or demand too much of them (Driscoll, 1981, 1989). At heart, these persons believe they are not capable of undertaking very much, and the prospect of others holding them responsible or expecting a great deal from them is quite frightening. If they communicate their inferiorities and incapabilities by publicly criticizing themselves, however, they might avert the danger by causing others to lower their expectations. This general strategy was colorfully portrayed by Eric Berne (1964) as the "game" of "Wooden Leg." This is a self-handicapping strategy (Berglas & Jones, 1978; Higgins et al., 1990; Snyder & Smith, 1982), in which persons diminish the expectations of others with pleas of the general form, "What do you expect of a person with a wooden leg?" (p. 160).

To Maintain Group Loyalty and Membership

To be a true member of any cohesive group and to maintain genuine loyalty and solidarity with others in it, one must subscribe to its core values, beliefs, and practices (Putman, 1990). However, on occasion, such subscription will entail engagement in rather destructive forms of self-appraisal, resulting in a situation where the price of belonging is self-mistreatment (Driscoll, 1984). For example, one client of mine belonged to a church that had as a core tenet the view that persons were inherently depraved sinners. As this person expressed the matter repeatedly to me, "My righteousness is as filthy rags in the eyes of the Lord." Essentially, he was in a situation where loyalty and belongingness with his church group required that he criticize himself as an abject, depraved, inherently sinful being.

Many individuals must criticize themselves in destructive ways if they are to remain loyal members of their own families (Driscoll, 1981, 1989; McKay & Fanning, 1992). Growing up, if they had rejected perfectionistic or other problematic standards, or if they had objected to the legitimacy of damaging parental criticism, this would have been regarded as a disrespectful refusal of parental authority. It would have constituted breaking rank with the family—refusing to be one of them and one with them by refusing to maintain allegiance to their core values and practices. For many persons, this familial situation does not change with the passage of time. As adults, it remains important to be a "good Smith" or a "loyal Jones." To be this, they must maintain allegiance to destructive standards and means of enforcement, no matter how damaging these may be to themselves.

SUMMARY

Many common purposes that persons are trying to accomplish by destructively criticizing themselves have been delineated in this section. These have included goals of improving themselves, avoiding egotism, atoning for past wrongs, maintaining a needed sense of superiority, protecting themselves from various dangers, diminishing the demands and expectations of others, expressing hostility, securing reassurance and sympathy, and maintaining group loyalty. As a rule, clients will be found to be pursuing several of these goals simultaneously. Assessing such purposes in collaboration with them helps them to own their self-critical behaviors, to examine their operating premises that these behaviors will achieve their desired ends, and to explore other more constructive modes of self-criticism that might better accomplish their goals.

ASSESSING SITUATIONS IN WHICH CLIENTS ARE MOST PRONE TO CRITICIZE THEMSELVES DESTRUCTIVELY

There are a number of life situations that tend, on a recurring basis, to stimulate self-critical persons to engage in especially severe attacks on themselves (Stone & Stone, 1993). In any person's life, his or her imperfect relationships, deeds, traits, skills, physical characteristics, and more can and often do provide a steady supply of grounds for destructive self-criticism. However, the situations of interest here tend more than most to exacerbate individuals' proclivities to attack themselves vigorously, and thus to engender more than the usual amounts of depression, anxiety, and diminished self-esteem. For this reason, it becomes important to assess such situations with clients. If they can become more aware of these danger points and of precisely how they respond to them as self-critics, the possibility is created that they can refrain from these customary behaviors and substitute more constructive alternatives. The following sections relate some of the situations that recurrently seem to result in especially vigorous self-critical attacks.

RECEPTION OF CRITICISM FROM OTHERS

Frequently, debilitating self-critical attacks are triggered by the subtle and not so subtle negative judgments of others (McKay &

Fanning, 1992; Stone & Stone, 1993). A parent, perhaps continuing an old refrain dating back to childhood, harshly attacks his grown daughter for being self-indulgent and spoiled. One friend criticizes another, perhaps subtly and with an overt aura of support and sympathy, for her failure to be strict enough with her son. A boss asks an employee how a certain piece of work is coming along, but with the underlying implication that it should have been done long ago.

As noted in previous chapters in a different connection, such external criticism is often especially devastating to individuals who are destructive critics of themselves. The latter have little defense against such judgments because they tend to concur automatically with them. Some of these persons simply conclude that they are "guilty as charged." Further, even when the matter might not be a "federal offense" for the external judge, with all sorts of global implications bearing on their basic worth, they will often view it as such an offense. The net effect will be that these persons will report such things as being "crushed" or "devastated" by external criticism and brooding about it for long periods of time. Later, in Chapter 7, specific therapeutic strategies for altering this reflexive pattern of concurrence will be related.

Other destructively self-critical persons have a different reaction to external criticism. They too at heart concur with their detractors, but their immediate reaction is to lash back very strongly at them (McKay & Fanning, 1992). Sensing their own vulnerability and sensing the pain, danger, or degradation inherent in going along with their critics, they counterattack quickly and strongly in the face of others' negative judgments. For this reason, they will be seen as "hypersensitive," "touchy," and "unable to take criticism." Essentially, these persons are trying to avert the kind of devastation that comes with simply capitulating to the indictments of others.

BEING IN THE PRESENCE OF CERTAIN OTHERS

Many individuals will report that their self-critical ways will be greatly exacerbated after contacts with certain other persons in their lives (Stone & Stone, 1993). The most infamous of such others tend to be the individual's parents or other family members, and for this reason family visits will tend to leave people depressed and feeling badly about themselves. Others who provoke such reactions may include certain friends, ex-spouses, bosses, enemies, or even mere acquaintances.

The avenues through which such others tend to potentiate especially severe self-critical attacks will vary. The first of them has already been discussed in the previous section: these other persons will be highly critical of the individual in direct or indirect ways. The second avenue has to do with other people having certain characteristics that tend to engender strong negative comparisons in the self-critical individual. The other person here does not have to *do* anything. Just being who he or she is provides grounds for self-criticism. For example, the other person might appear extremely self-assured, brilliant, highly achieving, physically attractive, interpersonally charismatic, or gifted in attracting romantic partners. The self-critical individual, perceiving such characteristics, turns on self with severe indictments of the general form, "Compared to _____, you are so utterly deficient."

The third avenue may sometimes be difficult to distinguish from the second. The impressive others that trigger critic attacks may not be simply being themselves. They may be engaging in very subtle competitive behavior—striving in perhaps skillfully unobtrusive ways to best others with their brilliance, beauty, charm, accomplishments, or social connections. The outcome here will be similar to that just mentioned. Such behavior will tend to stimulate destructively self-critical comparison behavior, but perhaps with more of a painful tinge of just having had one's nose rubbed in the dirt.

Major Failures and Setbacks

Significant failures and setbacks such as being rejected by a spouse or lover, losing one's job, flunking out of school, or failing to secure a prized position or relationship will tend to trigger particularly severe bouts of self-criticism (Stone & Stone, 1993; cf. Beck et al., 1979, on the manner in which negative life events activate depressogenic thinking). For example, Larry, a computer programmer in his middle thirties, came to therapy extremely depressed after his affections for a woman were not returned, and she began a new romantic relationship with another. In the wake of this, he experienced normal feelings of disappointment and grief. However, these "normal miseries of life" were compounded by the critical stance he adopted toward himself. He was absolutely furious with himself, denounced himself as a "fool" and as "sick" for permitting himself once again to become attached to someone who could not return his affections, told himself to "snap out of it and quit being so melodramatic" about his grief, and concluded that he was doomed never to find love. This hostile, degrading, and utterly unsympathetic reaction to loss resulted in Larry becoming suicidal. It typifies the way in which important failures and setbacks may stimulate especially severe self-critical behavior.

STRESSFUL SITUATIONS IN GENERAL

Stressful situations as a class are ones in which individuals are confronted with circumstances where it is vital to their interests that they succeed, but they have significant doubts that they possess the wherewithal (knowledge, skills, resources, physical attributes) to do so (cf. Lazarus, 1966; Lazarus & Folkman, 1984). Examples of persons in such stressful situations include students who have so many tests on one day that they are not sure they can succeed, airline flight controllers who must keep track of more planes aloft than they are sure they can manage, and single parents who are unsure they can manage the constant, myriad demands of their situation.

In the lives of destructively self-critical persons, stressful circumstances assume a wide and typical variety of forms. They might include difficulties in marital relationships, problems with children, or conflicts with employers. They might be normative family life crises such as marriage, the birth of a first child, the onset of adolescence, or the departure of a child from home (Carter & McGoldrick, 1989; Goldenberg & Goldenberg, 1991). They might entail being in new circumstances where one's well-established knowledge and competencies are believed insufficient, such as travel to a foreign country, taking on a new job, or entering a new academic program.

Destructively self-critical persons tend to become more self-critical under stressful circumstances (Stone & Stone, 1993). Such situations provide especially potent ammunition for them for two reasons. First, the likelihood of actual failures, mistakes, and less than optimum performance is much greater. Thus, there are simply more problematic things that the critic can target. Second, such situations engender anxiety and its usual accompaniments such as inability to concentrate, feelings of "not having it all together," and senses of "not being on top of things." Indeed, because many of these individuals have undermined their sense of self-efficacy through years of self-denigration, these anxiety symptoms will tend to be unusually severe. Frequently, this anxiety and these symptoms will themselves become grounds for further self-criticism ("What's wrong with me; I should just stop all of this quivering, get a grip, and get on top of this business!").

LOSS OF CONTROL IN SENSITIVE AREAS

Many persons have very sensitive areas in their lives where they strive mightily to maintain control and where they regard failures to do so as especially abhorrent and mortifying (Stone & Stone, 1993). For some persons, especially men, this might be strength and decisiveness; any vacillating or nonassertive behavior on their part that could seen as "weak" or "wishy-washy" or "wimpy" would be grounds for severe self-criticism (as well as humiliation). For others, the sensitive area might be sexual modesty and propriety; relaxations of tight control such as flirting or dancing provocatively would be intolerable. For yet others, it might be maintaining self-control in general; blowing up angrily or becoming drunkenly unrestrained would be highly unacceptable for such persons. For these individuals, any lapses from the maintenance of tight control in these sensitive areas tends to bring very strong self-critical reactions. In part, this will be to "punish the crime" severely; in part, it will be to reinstate a desperately wanted self-control (cf. Marshall, 1991, on the self-punitive reactions of bulimic individuals subsequent to eating binges).

ASSESSING HISTORICAL INFLUENCES ON DESTRUCTIVE SELF-CRITICAL BEHAVIOR

The assessment of historical influences on an individual's self-critical behavior may be useful in many cases. It might, for example, serve to show clients how what they are doing makes sense given their past. This often enables them to question the continued need for the behavior and gives them a reassuring sense that their debilitating actions are not crazy or perverse (Raimy, 1975). By way of further example, historical assessment may reveal influences from various sorts of unfinished business from the past (see, e.g., case of William in Chapter 5); or it might enable people to recognize that the hypercritical parents they placed so much credence in had certain limitations or agendas that vastly diminished their objectivity.

With this in mind, some of the historical factors that are empirically most common in cases of pathological self-criticism will be discussed in this section. The first of these factors has to do with how clients acquired the content of their later self-indictments. The second concerns how they often have learned the forms of criticism that they have. The third has to do with cultural influences on individuals' self-critical practices.

FAMILIAL LABEL ASSIGNMENT

Degrading labels often have a family history. When individuals brand themselves repeatedly with the same degrading labels, it will often be observed that these labels echo ones assigned long ago to the individual in his or her family of origin (Beck et al., 1979; Bowen, 1966; McKay & Fanning, 1992; Rubin, 1975; cf. Cooley, 1902, and Mead, 1934, on "the looking-glass self").

For example, Marcy, a young woman who has been mentioned several times previously in this book, grew up with a father who explicitly pronounced her "stupid," "incompetent," and "emotionally unstable" countless times over the course of her childhood. Moreover, he consistently treated her as being a person with these characteristics. For example, seeing her as incapable of handling her own affairs and as emotionally vulnerable, he frequently overfunctioned for her by doing things like bailing her out of financial difficulties that she created. Unable to disbelieve him (Marcy is the woman who commented that when her father spoke it was "like God speaking"), she assimilated all of his characterizations into her self-concept. When she came to therapy as a young adult, she regarded them as unquestioned truths about her and attributed them to herself routinely in a highly automatic, reflexive way.

Marcy's situation here is prototypical. That is, it embodies many of the features that are usually present in the familial transmission of debilitating labels and statuses. First, it began to occur at a time when Marcy was very young and vulnerable (McKay & Fanning, 1992; Rubin, 1975). At this time, her father, a successful professional man, was a forceful and persuasive critic of how things were in the world. Marcy, like most children, was an immature and unschooled neophyte in such matters who quite naturally accepted her father's pronouncements without question. In addition to this, Marcy's father had a severe temper, and was given to launching devastating verbal attacks on his children. Because she was extremely frightened of his tirades, Marcy was all the more constrained to go along with him. Thus, for many years prior to assuming adult observer and critic competencies, Marcy had been listening with complete faith to the "voice of God" telling her about her place and value in the world.

The second prototypical factor in this case is that the mode of transmission of Marcy's labels or statuses was not merely verbal, but also behavioral. She was not only told she was incompetent, she was treated as an incompetent person. Actions not only can "speak louder than words," but their implications can be more difficult to combat. When one is called "incompetent," it is at least out there on the table in an obvious way to react against. However, when one is treated as incompetent (e.g., by a father who is bailing one out of a difficult situation), especially when one is a young and inexperienced observer, this will often prove more difficult to detect and therefore to fight. Vague misgivings (e.g., that one should be handling this difficult situation on one's own) are often not articulated consciously, and the individual winds up participating in a transaction wherein he or she has accepted the other's degrading status assignment. In Marcy's case, each time she let her father overfunction for her, she accepted a nonverbal status assignment to the effect that she was helpless and incompetent.

The third and final prototypical factor here is that Marcy, after years of verbal pronouncements and treatment consistent with these, assimilated the labels and statuses assigned by others into her self-concept. They became the bedrock, unquestioned truth about her place and value in the world—about "who she really was." Like many people in her situation, Marcy had never stepped back as an adult and employed her much greater cognitive abilities to question and to reconsider these old givens. When status-relevant events occurred, her automatic reaction was to attribute the old, unquestioned labels to herself ("This just shows once again what a weak, helpless, incompetent person I am").

FAMILIAL MODELING OF SELF-CRITICAL PRACTICES

The literature on observational learning attests to the vast range of behaviors that one person can acquire through observing another (Bandura, 1969, 1977, 1986). Where the acquisition of maladaptive behavior is concerned, this literature tells us that two unfortunate things happen all too frequently. First, such behavior is modeled for a child, perhaps countless times by others who meet with some success with its employment. Second, more adaptive alternative behaviors are either not available for the child to observe and acquire or, if they are present, are observed to meet with punishing or ineffectual consequences (Liebert & Spiegler, 1994). Thus, for example, children may become problematically aggressive by being exposed to models who are successful with inappropriately aggressive behavior and by not being exposed to models who are successful with skillful assertive or negotiating behaviors.

Viewed from this observational learning perspective, what too many individuals get during their developmental years are essentially lessons in how to criticize themselves in destructive ways. What they do not get are lessons in how to do so in constructive and beneficial ways (Frost, Lahart, & Rosenblat, 1991; Koestner, Zuroff, & Powers, 1991). Growing up in families where practices such as the attribution of degrading labels, the imposition of perfectionistic standards, and the employment of harshly punitive measures out of all proportion to offenses, individuals accumulate vast amounts of observation. They see their parents subjecting them, their siblings, and even each other to such treatment (Harris & Howard, 1984; Jaenicke, Hammen, Zupan, Hiroto, Gordon, Adrian, & Burge, 1987). They also may observe their parents subjecting themselves to it (Rubin, 1975). Further, they are exposed to peers, teachers, coaches, siblings, religious leaders and media figures who may also constitute potent models of critic functioning. Finally, what many children do not get to observe to any appreciable extent are others successfully employing benign and constructive critical practices.

Many authors, taking their cue from the landmark work of Freud (1923) (see also Brenner, 1974), describe the acquisition of self-critical behaviors as being the result of introjection or incorporation of the morally praising or prohibiting parent. For example, McKay and Fanning (1992, p. 19) state that, "His [the critic's] voice is the voice of a disapproving parent, the punishing, forbidding voice that shaped your behavior as a child." From the present point of view, such a way of talking is simply another acceptable way to say the same thing: that modes of criticism that one was subjected to previously by others have been observed, acquired, and personally accepted (internalized) as ways to criticize oneself.

An example of this process of acquisition occurred in the case of Dan, a highly successful media personality in his late thirties. Dan reported during the course of therapy that he found fault with everything he did and had ever done. He thus derived almost no personal satisfaction from his considerable professional and civic accomplishments. Further, he related, it was a matter of deliberate policy with him never to permit himself to be satisfied and always to think about how something could and should have been done better. He strongly believed that letting oneself be satisfied with an accomplishment was tantamount to becoming complacent and ceasing to strive for ever greater excellence. Such complacency was, in his mind, the first step on the road to mediocrity.

In discussing the origins of this pattern, Dan related that his father had never been satisfied with any of his accomplishments. His father had employed approval as a sort of "carrot" that was never given but always dangled just a bit out of his children's reach. No matter what Dan did, his father would always inquire why it had not been done just a little bit better. Further, he told Dan explicitly that he did not want to praise him for anything, because he was afraid that his son would then relax, become self-satisfied, and cease to strive for improvement. In Dan's case, the parental pattern of critical behavior, as well as the rationale behind it, had been imitated to the letter.

CULTURAL INFLUENCES ON SELF-CRITICAL BEHAVIOR

A set of influences that has shaped many clients historically, and continues to do so, comes from the broader culture (Barrow & Moore, 1983; Rubin, 1975). These influences take the form primarily of certain standards that get promulgated as criteria of personal adequacy. These standards are transmitted through countless, enormously pervasive sources. These include other persons such as individuals' parents, peer group members, siblings, teachers, coaches, and community leaders. They also include media sources such as television and radio programming, movies, books, and magazines (and the massive amounts of advertising emanating from these sources).

Among the more pernicious of such standards, the ones listed below seem most prominent. They are adapted from Rubin (1975, pp. 190–234), and the reader is referred to that source for an in-depth discussion. However, for purposes of economy, they will be condensed here into a simple set of "thou shalt nots" that are widely promulgated and espoused in American society.

1. Thou shalt not be unmarried or not in a committed relationship ("You're nobody 'til somebody loves you").
2. Thou shalt not be without notable vocational or other accomplishments, or be unsuccessful.
3. Thou shalt not be less than a winner in all of life's endeavors.

4. Thou shalt not be a member of a nonprestigious profession.
5. Thou shalt not be in the wrong position for one's gender (e.g., a male nurse or a female executive).
6. Thou shalt not be emotionally disturbed in any way.
7. Thou shalt not be physically handicapped.
8. Thou shalt not have certain physical illnesses (e.g., AIDS, herpes) (Pryor & Reeder, 1993).
9. Thou shalt not be sexually attracted to members of one's own gender.
10. Thou shalt not be possessed of nonnormative sexual appetites ("perverted").
11. Thou shalt not be physically unattractive.
12. Thou shalt not be short.
13. Thou shalt not be overweight.
14. Thou shalt not be old.
15. Thou shalt not be nonwhite.
16. Thou shalt not be indecisive (a "wimp," "wishy-washy").
17. Thou shalt not be unpopular.
18. Thou shalt not be poor.
19. Thou shalt not be uneducated.
20. Thou shalt not be unintelligent.
21. Thou shalt not be anything less than endlessly striving for self-betterment ("being all that you can be").

Oftentimes, assessment reveals that these broad cultural standards have exercised, and continue to exercise, a profound effect on individuals. As critics of themselves, these persons have in effect been coopted by the society in these regards. Despite the blatant unfairness, discrimination, inhumanity, and/or impossibility inherent in them, these standards have been internalized. Thus, clients tell us that because they are unmarried, or homosexual, or without great accomplishments, they regard themselves as worthless. They experience these characteristics as stigmata (Goffman, 1963; Jones, Farina, Hastorf, Markus, Miller, & Scott, 1984) that disqualify them from being fully worthy, entitled members of society.

SUMMARY

When initial clinical exploration reveals that destructive self-critical behaviors are to be the target of intervention, a broad array of matters should be assessed. These include the precise nature of clients' self-critical behaviors, their sensed ownership of them, the purposes they are trying to accomplish with them, the situations that tend disproportionately to trigger them, and historical influences on them from familial and societal sources.

HELPING CLIENTS TO ABANDON PATHOLOGICAL SELF-CRITICAL PRACTICES

Some problems simply vanish when the attempted solution is correctly interdicted.

LYNN SEGAL (1991, p. 192)

In this chapter, a general strategy for helping persons to abandon pathological self-critical practices will be described. At times, the accomplishment of this objective is sufficient by itself for therapy to be terminated. The first domino has been tipped over, setting in motion a series of other positive changes, and therapy may end here with a highly satisfactory outcome. At other times, much attention must be paid to the accomplishment of a second objective, that of helping persons to acquire and to commit themselves to the use of more benign and constructive means of criticizing themselves. The latter will comprise the primary focus of the remainder of the book.

The central therapeutic intervention described in this chapter is a seemingly paradoxical one. In this intervention, clients are directed to continue their detrimental self-critical behaviors in certain carefully prescribed ways. Discussion of this intervention will include explications of the following: (1) the theoretical considerations that underly it; (2) some groundwork that should be done before the directive is given; (3) the precise nature of the directive itself; (4) follow-up procedures for clients who respond in various ways; (5) some hypotheses regarding the change principles involved; and (6) some suggestions for helping the many clients who change but then become frightened that they will regress.

THEORETICAL UNDERPINNINGS OF THE PRESENT STRATEGY

Two clinical theories guide the approach described in this chapter. These are the *status dynamic* position of Ossorio and his associates (Bergner, 1987, 1988, 1993; Ossorio, 1976, 1982; Schwartz, 1979; Wechsler, 1993) and the *second order change* position of Watzlawick and his associates (Fisch, Weakland, & Segal, 1982; Segal, 1991; Watzlawick, 1978, 1988; Watzlawick, Weakland, & Fisch, 1974). Both of these will be reviewed briefly.

Ossorio's Status Dynamic Position

This orientation is concerned with an individual's *status* as a crucial determinant of the range of actions in which he or she is able to participate. The status of a person is defined as the totality of his or her relationships with all the elements of the world (Ossorio, 1976, 1982; Shideler, 1988). The term thus designates an individual's overall position or place in the scheme of things. This position is divisible into any number of subrelationships. For example, the terms "father," "friend," "employee," "self-rejecter," "scapegoat," "outcast," "ally," "religious adherent," "sergeant," and "victim of discrimination" are among the countless positions that a given individual might occupy.

Critically, to occupy certain positions in relation to other persons, objects, states of affairs, or even oneself enhances one's freedom and ability to act (Bergner, 1987, 1988, 1993; Ossorio, 1976, 1982). To occupy other positions constricts such freedom and ability. For example, an individual in a military hierarchy might occupy the position of "private" or of "general." The mere occupation of the latter position by an individual carries with it a greatly expanded power and range of possible behaviors relative to the former. Furthermore, this behavior potential accrues to the occupant of this position independently of his or her beliefs, skills, motivations, traits, or other personal characteristics (although, of course, persons who differ in such regards will implement positions differently). Although the example of positions in a military hierarchy may make the point in an especially clear way, status dynamics emphasizes and exploits the fact that all positions or relationships convey varying degrees of behavior potential.

From the status dynamic perspective, the task of psychotherapy is status enhancement (Ossorio, 1976). That is, it is helping clients to occupy positions of enhanced power and/or eligibility from which they may act to achieve desired life goals. Frequently, this entails helping individuals to occupy new, more viable relational positions. Much of family therapy, for example, may be thought of as undertaking the task of helping individuals to occupy more viable interpersonal positions (e.g., to help young adults liberate themselves from their families of origin by extricating them from parentified, or scapegoated, or peacemaking roles). More frequently, the goal of therapy becomes that of helping individuals to realize relational positions that they already occupy but which, for whatever reason, they have failed to realize and to exploit.

Viewed from a status dynamic perspective, the great majority of clients who are pathological self-critics enter psychotherapy with a view of themselves as occupying the position or status of victim. As noted in previous chapters, they see themselves as helplessly in the grips of such states of affairs as depression, anxiety, low self-esteem, mental illness, and extreme vulnerability to critical persons in their lives. Status dynamic theory heuristically suggests that such persons might best be helped first by enabling them to recognize that they occupy an infinitely more powerful position vis-à-vis their problems—that of perpetrator of destructively self-critical behaviors. It also suggests that these persons might then be assisted further by showing them how they can capitalize on this far more powerful position to bring about meaningful change.

THE SECOND-ORDER CHANGE PERSPECTIVE

The second-order change perspective has emerged from theoretical and empirical work done over many years at the Mental Research Institute in Palo Alto, California (Fisch et al., 1982; Segal, 1991; Watzlawick, 1978, 1988; Watzlawick et al., 1974). The originators of this theoretical orientation have focused their primary attention on clients' tendencies to erect certain kinds of commonsense formulations of the nature of their problems. Unfortunately, when these formulations are used to generate solutions and then to implement them, clients tend to engage in behaviors that serve to maintain and perpetuate, rather than to solve, the problem. This is so because these individuals make change attempts only within the parameters of the inadequate problem formulation (first-order change), in a situation where meaningful change requires transcendance of or escape from these parameters (second-order change).

An interesting example of such problem formulations and solution attempts may be found in the anthropologist Carlos Castaneda's account of his apprenticeship to the Indian sorcerer Don Juan (Castaneda, 1968, 1972, 1974). At one point, Carlos and Don Juan take up the matter of the former's competitive orientation to other people. Carlos conceives all of his interpersonal encounters as contests from which he emerges either a winner or a loser (Castaneda, 1972, pp. 122–129). Believing himself too often the loser, the only form of change he can envision is that he become a winner. This formulation dooms Carlos to first-order change attempts. His predicament is that even if he changes in the only way his formulation permits him to envision (i.e., by "winning" more of his interpersonal encounters), he remains enmeshed in a thoroughly competitive orientation to human relationships. He continues to miss out on the satisfactions inherent in other, noncompetitive ways of relating to others. In a very real sense, even if he wins, he loses.

The task of the therapist, from this theoretical perspective, is that he or she help clients to engage in second-order change attempts. In such attempts, clients cease to operate within the constraints imposed by their commonsense problem formulations. Instead, they act on the basis of reformulations that permit them to escape or transcend these constraints. In the example cited, Don Juan attempts to help Carlos toward second-order change by, among other things, instructing him to "see like a crow" (Castaneda, 1972, p. 122). Explaining this puzzling directive, Don Juan relates that the crow has a noncompetitive relationship with other elements of the world. The crow never contests with other animals, but spends its life seeking that which is pleasing. Rather than watching Carlos thrash about in his "winner–loser" quandary, Don Juan instructs him at length in how to see like a crow. Furthermore, he guides him in gaining experience in this very different, far more hedonically oriented mode of choosing and behaving (see Farber, 1981, for a fascinating account of Don Juan's change tactics).

Viewed from the second-order change perspective, destructively self-critical actions may be seen often as first-order change attempts. Guided by commonsense formulations of their problems in living, persons have concluded that criticizing themselves in certain ways represent solutions to their difficulties (cf. Chapter 3 discussion of purposes of self-criticism). For example, they may have conceived their problems with depression and low self-esteem as due to their historically inadequate achievements, and thus generated the solution of engaging in ever more strenuous attempts to "crack the whip" and get themselves in line. Or, in the face of a history replete with scorn and degradation from others, they may have come to see the only satisfying solution as one of achieving a narcissistic triumph over their detractors. Of course, "showing them" requires that one be a superior being, and achieving such superiority will require considerable resort to the imposition of superhuman standards. These self-critical clients typically come to therapy when their solution attempts have not worked and indeed are maintaining the depression, low self-esteem, and other problems that they were designed to relieve. What such persons need from the therapist, more than anything else, is a new formulation of their problem that will enable them to escape or transcend the restrictions imposed by their present ones. The "perpetrator of destructive self-criticism" formulation is one that can provide them access to second-order change attempts and ultimately success.

LAYING THE GROUNDWORK FOR THE THERAPEUTIC DIRECTIVE

MINIMIZING RESISTANCE

A potentially powerful directive is useless if the client resists or rejects it. Thus, an important subgoal in the present strategy becomes that of presenting such directives to clients in ways that maximize the probability of their compliance. For the author, the following ideas have proven most effective in this regard.

Appeal to What Matters

This policy suggests that therapeutic efforts in general, and here directives in particular, be aligned with the clients' existing motivations (Driscoll, 1984; Fisch et al., 1982; Ossorio, 1976). Rather than declaring certain clients "unmotivated," or appealing to motives that, however commendable, they do not possess, the suggestion is that the therapist assess clients' *actual* motivations. Apprised of these, he or she should then frame directives in such a way that clients see their implementation as consistent with their existing motivations. Thus, if moral considerations are paramount for certain individuals, we are relatively unlikely to be successful by urging such persons to "give up their shoulds." We are more likely to be successful by portraying old behavior as in some way contrary to the person's moral values and new behavior as in some way consistent with those values. Similarly, persons who value highly such things as personal strength, independence, control, integrity, being different, or being logical may best be approached in ways that are consistent with their existing values.

In the present context, this policy suggests that great care be taken by the therapist not to frame the basic directive in such a way that it seems to violate the client's values and/or to entail a renunciation of cherished goals. In contrast, the framing should be such that its compatibility with existing values and goals is stressed to the degree that this is possible.

The "Positive Connotation"

The Milan Associates (Selvini-Palazzoli, Boscolo, Cecchin, & Prata, 1978; Selvini-Palazzoli, Cirillo, & Selvini, 1989) have reported that reframes and associated directives are accepted more readily when problematic behavior is given a "positive connotation." By this, they mean that the behavior is portrayed in some desirable or commendable fashion. For example, with respect to self-critical behaviors, framings in which the person is portrayed as engaging in attempts at "self-improvement," the "pursuit of excellence," or the "avoidance of conceit" are in general more likely to be accepted than ones wherein the person is portrayed as "ridden with irrational shoulds," "perfectionistic," or "masochistic."

Speaking to the Client's "Position"

Second-order change theorists (Fisch et al., 1982; Segal, 1991; Watzlawick et al., 1974) have advocated that therapists consider the client's entire "position" and custom tailor all reframes and directives in light of this. The client's position comprises such things as his or her (1) current view of the problem (e.g., is it seen as "sickness" or as "badness"); (2) characteristic language (e.g., visual language such as "my view is . . ."); (3) favored metaphors (e.g., gambling ones such as "seems like a long shot"); (4) personal characteristics (e.g., religiosity or altruism); (5) values (e.g., for achievement or good relationships); and (6) what he or she is seeking from the therapist (e.g., insight, support, or concrete suggestions). In general, the policy here is to see that all reframes and directives are carefully designed so that they fit as well as possible with the person's overall position, and thus make it maximally likely that they will be accepted.

PLANNING

A considerable amount of planning must go into the creation of a custom-tailored directive for clients (Fisch et al., 1982). A great deal of information is reflected in the decision as to what precise form it should take and how exactly it should be framed or "packaged" for the client. To summarize briefly what has been said in this chapter and the last, the following elements should have been assessed and should be reflected in the final prescription. First, the precise nature of the target self-critical practices should be known. Second, some sense of ownership of these behaviors should have been established; clients should be exhibiting at a minimum a recognition that they are the authors of self-directed critical actions. Third, clients' primary purposes or goals for self-critical behaviors should have been ascertained to a fair degree; are they seeking self-improvement, safety from external criticism, a sense of themselves as very special, or other specific goals? Fourth, if the actions in question tend to occur primarily in one certain situation, this should be determined. Fifth, the individual's values and general position as characterized above should be known. Sixth and finally, relevant historical influences, especially ones that shed some light on current maintaining factors, should have been ascertained.

In planning the directive, the ideal (if rarely actual) state of affairs would be that it reflect all of the above elements and that it not violate any of them (e.g., be seen as antithetical to a cherished goal or value of the client). Where certain of these elements prove difficult to establish, the directive should not be implemented unless and until they are established. Most importantly, if clients cannot identify with reasonable precision their self-critical acts, or if they are highly resistant or unable to acknowledge that they are their perpetrators, the directive should not (indeed cannot) be utilized.

THE DIRECTIVE: PRESCRIBING DESTRUCTIVE SELF-CRITICAL BEHAVIOR

The following therapeutic procedure is one of the most powerful mentioned in this book. When the groundwork assessment and planning measures discussed above have been executed carefully, it often achieves sudden and far-reaching changes in a relatively short period of time. Reduced to its essentials, the procedure may be stated simply: it consists in recommending to clients that they continue to engage in their problematic self-critical behaviors consciously and deliberately. Now that they have recognized how they function as critics of themselves and their purposes in doing so, they are urged to continue to do as they have been doing, but to do so intentionally and with full awareness.

An example of such a prescription might serve best to convey the nature of this strategy. "Right now," it might be suggested to a client, "you have told me that you have always imposed very perfectionistic standards upon yourself, and you have detailed exactly how you do this. Despite all of the pain, frustration, and constant sense of failure that this has produced, you have felt that you must treat yourself this way for fear that, if you did not, you would wind up a complacent mediocrity, despised and disrespected by others. To date, you have done all of this almost reflexively; you have become so good at it that you can carry it out on automatic pilot largely outside of your own awareness. In the coming week, I would like to suggest something that may surprise you: that you continue to do precisely what you have been doing—that you continue to impose those perfectionistic standards exactly as you have been—but that you take this behavior off of automatic pilot and engage in it consciously and deliberately."

In the present approach, the goal of this directive is *not* the manipulative and paradoxical one of rendering the client immediately unable to do as he or she has been doing. It is the more existential goal of helping persons to responsibly own, take control of, and ultimately have a choice with respect to their problematic behavior. It is the goal of helping persons to occupy positions of enhanced power from which they may act to improve their lives (Bergner, 1993).

RATIONALIZING THE PRESCRIPTION TO CLIENTS

A critical part of this prescription lies in the provision of rationales to individuals regarding why they should engage consciously and deliberately in behavior already acknowledged to be destructive and why they should in effect restrain themselves from trying to change immediately. This is critical for two reasons. First, it has been noted by previous authors (e.g., Fisch et al., 1982; Hoffman, 1981) that, if one is going to engage in the seemingly nonsensical act of directing persons to continue with problematic behaviors, one must provide some strong rationale for them to do so. One must buttress apparent nonsense with sense. Second, in contrast with "symptom-prescribing" approaches, these rationales are not just cover stories designed to disguise the real, paradoxical intents of the therapist. They can and should contain the actual rationales and reasons why the therapist is advocating deliberate enactment of problematic behaviors. The primary rationales utilized by the author to encourage clients to deliberately perpetrate destructive self-critical behaviors are described in the following sections.

Rationale: "It Will Help You to Gain Control"

Clients may be informed that engaging in their problematic self-critical behaviors consciously and deliberately will help them to gain control over them. "Right now," they may be told, "you are on 'automatic pilot' with respect to your self-critical actions. You engage in them reflexively, with very little awareness, and therefore little control. Doing them on purpose will take them off of automatic pilot, will help you to take greater personal control over them, will give you a great deal more awareness, and ultimately will give you a whole lot more choice in the matter of whether you want to continue or discontinue these actions."

Rationale: "Appreciate Your Positive Reasons"

By the time the present directive is utilized, clients will already be aware that they are behaving in self-critical ways because they have some good reasons to do so. With this in mind, they might be reminded that to attempt to instantaneously drop their self-critical practices is to run the danger of trying to disregard these good reasons. However, these reasons will not go away, and trying to pretend they don't exist cannot work. "Therefore," a typical directive might go, "I would like to suggest that you keep doing as you are doing this week but pay a whole lot of attention to *why* you are doing it. What are you trying to accomplish with the behavior? Are you accomplishing it? Do you derive any satisfactions from the behavior? Consider what life would be like if you ceased the behavior—do you get any sense that this would be a loss or that there might be some danger if you stopped? Please note *any* reason that occurs to you, even if you are not sure about it. A lot of these reasons, I think you'll continue to find, are good ones, and you may decide that despite the personal costs you should not change. However, if you do decide to change, it would be advisable for you to be aware of your good reasons so that you can incorporate them into any changes you might wish to make."

Rationale: "Appreciate Your Reasons to Discontinue"

As a rule, clients are quite aware of reasons to discontinue maladaptive self-critical behaviors. They are aware of the personal pain, interpersonal difficulties, and other disadvantages created by these behaviors. However, sometimes they are not aware of these costs. In these cases, an indicated suggestion is to continue to behave as they have been, but to notice the costs and disadvantages of doing so. For example, many persons who are highly judgmental of others fail to appreciate that their critical ways are a two-edged sword that is turned not only on others but on themselves as well (Bergner, 1981). Thus, they are minimally aware of reasons they might have to discontinue such a harshly prosecutorial approach to the world.

Rationale: "Never Trust Overnight Changes"

Clients may be informed that, appealing as the prospect might be, it is extremely unlikely that they can jump instantaneously from a long-practiced, habitual way of criticizing themselves to its diametric opposite or complete elimination. Further, even if they did manage to do so, the permanence of the change would be suspect. It would rest on an impulsive decision made without giving full and careful consideration to important relevant matters and without listening to and respecting one's feelings of reluctance to change. In contrast, the conservative approach of continuing to enact self-critical behaviors deliberately, while giving careful consideration to the sorts of reasons mentioned above, is a way to proceed slowly and responsibly toward a decision that will rest on a much firmer foundation.

FOLLOW-UP MEASURES

Clients typically react to prescriptions to continue their self-critical behaviors in one of three ways. The first and empirically least common of these ways is that they ignore or disregard them. Here, they do not truly engage the directive in the sense of actively refusing or actively complying with its content. Occasionally, such clients seem startlingly oblivious to the fact that a directive had even been given the previous week. In any event, the suggested response to such a dismissive reaction is to investigate what happened. Was the client aware of the directive? Did he or she have an adverse reaction to it? What precisely happened that resulted in its being set aside? Depending on the outcome of this inquiry, the therapeutic decision may be made to issue the directive again or to drop it and utilize other avenues to change, including other modes of giving homework assignments (see DeShazer, 1984, 1985, on adjusting future directives in light of clients' responses to earlier ones).

The second response to the prescription to continue destructive self-critical patterns is an active refusal to do so. Here, clients cease their engagement in these debilitating practices, and consequently report feeling considerably better. However, such refusals will frequently entail a fearful avoidance of the self-critical behaviors and so less of a sense of ultimate ownership and control. For this reason, the suggested therapeutic response to such refusal is to attempt one additional time to secure compliance with the directive. In the author's experience, even when the client again does not comply, this additional refusal seems to solidify the therapeutic gain.

The third and most therapeutically desirable response to the directive to continue self-critical actions is that clients implement it. They return saying things like, "I tried what you suggested," and go on to report good faith efforts to implement the prescription. In response to such compliance, recommended follow-up moves include (1) expressing appreciation for their efforts, (2) asking for a careful report on what they observed when they engaged in their problematic behaviors on purpose, (3) underscoring any new sense of control over critic behaviors exhibited by the client, and (4) exploring the results of self-monitoring aspects of the directive (e.g., "Did it seem like treating yourself this way last week led to self-improvement or not?"). In a somewhat unconventional way, these sessions become insight therapy sessions in which such things as the objectives of the behavior, any satisfactions inherent in it, and any fears of what would ensue if the behavior changed are all brought to conscious awareness and explicitly discussed. Finally, clients are encouraged to continue perpetrating the behavior for one or two additional weeks and urged to gather further observations each week. Subsequent sessions continue to assume the form just described.

The results of successful compliance with this directive are typically greater senses of ownership and control over the critic behaviors, and thus an enhanced sense of choice in the matter of whether or not to abandon them. Most clients who attempt to comply and meet with reasonable success in their attempts to take control of maladaptive critic behaviors abandon these actions in a period ranging from several days to several weeks. Their most common report is that they cannot continue to perpetrate such behaviors consciously and deliberately once they have appreciated fully the exact nature and consequences of what they have been doing to themselves. Often, they will report that, even when they were doing them consciously and deliberately, they found themselves unable to take what they were doing "seriously." Further, in some cases clients will spontaneously generate more benign and constructive ways to criticize themselves. Somewhat more frequently, the therapist will need to provide assistance in generating such alternatives (see Chapters 6 and 7).

Occasionally, individuals comply with the directive to engage deliberately in maladaptive critic behaviors, but do not cease to enact them. Further inquiry reveals that the original formulation of the problem was adequate and that the client has achieved both good understanding and good control of the behavior. In such cases, the client has shifted to an existential position in which he or she is choosing to maintain the problematic self-critical behaviors. In such circumstances, the therapist should shift to the sorts of therapeutic measures mentioned in subsequent chapters, while consistently approaching and treating the client as one who occupies the high-power perpetrator position. The prevailing existential question, implicit always in the modes of speech employed, in the "angle" from which the problem is attacked, and in any future directives given is always, "Do you wish or not wish to continue this mode of self-critical behavior?" (Bergner, 1993).

Ultimately, a very few persons will elect, after compliance with the present directive and subsequent very thorough work on this issue, to continue their self-destructive practices. The recommended position of the therapist toward such clients is the following: "You have come to a position where you are very clear on what you are doing as a critic. You are no longer on 'automatic pilot' but are in charge of this behavior. You no longer live with the sense that the pain and difficulties that it creates are mysteriously and uncontrollably visited upon you, but are fully aware that you are behaving in a way that carries these costs. Further, you have decided that you are willing to incur these costs in the interests of obtaining the benefits of your behavior. This is no longer a psychological problem; it is a mature choice." Such clients, with respect to their critic behaviors, are left in this position and are not urged further to change. From here, they are ideally positioned to redecide the matter at a later date should they desire to do so.

TWO CASE ILLUSTRATIONS

THE CASE OF WILLIAM

William, a highly intelligent, 32-year-old doctoral candidate in English literature, made a rather dramatic appearance at intake. Wearing a long dark cape, a dark, brooding look, and long, disheveled hair, the first impression he created was that he had just walked off the stage from playing Hamlet. During his initial therapy session, William stated that he suffered from "anhedonia." Substantiating this unusual problem description, he reported that he found himself substantially unable to derive pleasure or meaning from his graduate studies, his work as a teaching assistant, or his relationship with his girlfriend, even though all of these seemed to him in some objective sense to be proceeding well. William had done some reading in psychology and conceived his anhedonia as a "symptom." He believed that it represented the outward manifestation of something within him that he could not comprehend and therefore could not control. This view had left him vacillating for 12 years between two basic modes of behavior: (1) attempting to achieve insight into these underlying factors, and (2) despairing and doing nothing. When seen, he had substantially concluded that the achievement of pleasure and meaning were beyond his control.

Exploration of William's personal history revealed that, as a child and adolescent, he had experienced a great deal of disparagement and humiliation at the hands of both his family and his peers, the details of which need not be related here. William's response to this degrading treatment was to resolve that one day he would "show them all." As his inclinations and talents developed over the years, the form that this "showing them" assumed was that he would write a great novel that would be hailed universally by critics. In the wake of this accomplishment, he would win all manner of prestigious literary prizes, appear on the cover of *Time* magazine, and become a famous American literary figure. Then, all of his former degraders and tormentors would realize that they had completely misjudged him and would bitterly regret that they could not bask now in his reflected glory. In one of his fantasies, persons from his past would come to him and ask him if he remembered them.

He would look at them in a bored and disinterested way and dismissively reply that, "No, I'm afraid I don't; now if you would excuse me, I'm terribly busy."

After hearing in considerable detail the above description, William's therapist, drawing upon an interest that William had stated in Platonic philosophy, commented that William's desired scenario reminded him of a Platonic idea. That is, for William, the idea of this triumphant scenario—this scenario of total acclamation, vindication, and revenge over his childhood tormentors—served as an ideal. Relative to this ideal, all actual activities, relationships, and accomplishments were being judged by him to be but pale, unfulfilling approximations. On considering this description, William agreed that indeed this seemed to be the case.

The therapist then gave William a directive to deliberately engage in what amounted to a caricature version of his self-critical actions. He suggested to William that he set aside five minutes per day for the following week. During this five minutes, he was to close his eyes and to completely indulge himself in the fantasy and the attendant satisfactions of his perfect triumph and vindication. At the end of this five minutes, he was to open his eyes and to say aloud with conviction: "Compared to this, I *declare* every other activity and accomplishment worthless and meaningless."

A week later, William returned to therapy. He reported that he had followed the directive for three days, but on the fourth day discontinued it because "it no longer seemed relevant." The problem, he stated, was "ancient history" for him inasmuch as he had ceased as a critic to disqualify his everyday activities, accomplishments, and relationships, and so he felt no need to continue. Subsequent discussion revealed that William in fact was deriving far more meaning and satisfaction from his life at this time. While further therapeutic work regarding this and other problems ensued, the above episode proved a decisive turning point in William's ultimately successful therapy.

THE CASE OF MICHAEL

Michael, the 35-year-old married graphic artist who was mentioned in Chapter 3, reported in therapy that he would often become quite depressed and dissatisfied with himself after attending social gatherings. Queried about what exactly seemed to be happening at these gatherings, Michael related that his problems would typically occur if there was some other male in attendance whom he found to be very impressive. When this happened, he would always compare himself with the other man, come out a poor second best, and emerge feeling quite depressed and inferior (cf. work on "upward social comparison" by Wills, 1986, and Wheeler & Miyake, 1992).

On getting this general picture, the therapist asked Michael to "give me a lesson in precisely what I would have to do if I wanted to go from simply noticing an impressive man to becoming very depressed; please direct me regarding what specific steps I would have to take to do this to myself." The purpose of this directive was to attempt to do two things at once. The first was to assess Michael's self-critical behavior, so that both he and the therapist would be aware of the precise actions involved. The second was to get him to describe it in deliberate action language (e.g., "Well, the first thing you would have to do is . . ."). In effect, the aim was to get Michael to reframe this comparison problem for himself, not as something that happened to him, but as something he did (and, by implication, could refrain from doing).

Michael was agreeable to providing the requested "lesson." He stated that the first "step" was to notice another male who was in some respect quite impressive. The most recent example had been a man who was noted locally for his athletic prowess. The therapist inquired whether or not the man had to be noteworthy in some way that was important in terms of Michael's values. In response to this inquiry, Michael smiled in a somewhat sheepish but good-natured way, as if to say, "Now that I make it explicit, I can't believe I do this silly thing." He indicated that many of the men's virtues, including the most recent one of athleticism, were actually very low on his own scale of values. Step two in the lesson thus became: "Disregard your own values and adopt the other individual's."

Asked about step three, Michael stated that this entailed comparing himself to the other man and finding himself inferior. Again the therapist called for a clarification: Did Michael engage in an overall comparison of the other fellow's strong and weak points with his own strong and weak points? Smiling again, Michael related that he singled out only the other's outstanding positive characteristic and compared himself only in that regard. Thus, step three became: "Compare yourself to the other individual, focusing *only* on his outstanding characteristic; deliberately disregard both his weak points and your own strengths."

Proceeding, Michael said that step four consisted in berating himself for his inferiority with respect to the target characteristic.

This consisted in an essentially reflexive action of equating being inferior in this respect with being defective as a person. One of his favorite self-characterizations was that it meant he was an "—hole." Step four thus became: "Tell yourself that because you are inferior to this man in X respect, even though X may be low on your scale of values, you are an —hole."

Michael related that step five depended on whether or not the desired change was possible or impossible for him. If possible, he would devise a personal plan for self-improvement in the target area. Step six would then consist in implementing that plan for about a week, at which time he would usually give it up. If the improvement in question was judged impossible, he related, step five would be "just feel miserable."

In the course of Michael's recitation, the therapist recorded the steps on a note card in deliberate action language, much in the way they have been characterized above in quotation marks. At the conclusion, the note card was handed to Michael, along with a directive and rationale along the following general lines: "Right now, Michael, you can do this comparison number in your sleep, it's so automatic. To get control over it, it's important to get it off of autopilot so that you can choose to do it or not do it in the future. For this reason, I'd like to suggest that you take this card with you, keep it in your wallet, and if you go to a party, take it out and consciously and deliberately run through these steps. Maybe you could slip off to the bathroom to do it. Then, why don't you come back in two weeks and report to me exactly what you've done and what you observed." Michael agreed, although still with a self-deprecatingly humorous attitude that seemed to say: "I can't believe what I just said; it seems so silly when you spell it out explicitly." He returned two weeks later stating that, even though he had an opportunity, he found himself unable to take the steps seriously any more, now that he was aware of what exactly he was doing. In the ensuing months of the therapy, he reported no further problems with this destructively self-critical comparison scenario.

CHANGE PRINCIPLES

Why do clients often cease to enact their destructive self-critical behaviors in the context of the present strategy? Indeed, to place this question in a larger context, why in general do "restraint from change" techniques seem to work (Fisch et al., 1982; Hoffman, 1981; Weeks & L'Abate, 1982)? The following explanatory change principles represent the author's hypotheses regarding the solution to this question.

CLIENT HAS SHIFTED TO POSITION OF CONTROL

When all proceeds according to plan in the present strategy, the client makes a radical positional shift. His or her initial position is the very low-power one comprising (1) not realizing how one is functioning as a critic, (2) genuinely conceiving self as victimized and therefore helpless, and (3) holding a problem formulation that renders solution impossible. The client's final position is the high-power one comprising (1) knowing what one is doing as a self-critic to create the problem; (2) doing this in a conscious, deliberate, and planful way, and (3) fully appreciating one's reasons to continue or discontinue these actions. In this final position, the behavior is into awareness and off of "automatic pilot." The client is actively choosing, is responsibly owning, and is in charge of the very behavior that is causing the difficulties. The client knows what he or she is choosing and why. This is a position, as status dynamic theory would highlight, from which the choice may also be made to cease the behavior. This is a problem formulation, as second-order change theory would highlight, from which old solution attempts can be interdicted and new, more adequate ones can be generated.

NEUTRALIZATION OF UNHELPFUL SELF-COERCION

Frequently, when clients realize what they are doing to themselves as critics, their initial reaction is, "I must stop doing these destructive things to myself." They place an immediate, coercive pressure on themselves to cease. This self-coercive "reflex" disregards their reasons for doing as they are doing, their right to consider these reasons, and their right to make a true personal choice. Thus, it typically elicits resistance from self, which here takes the form of refusing to relinquish the maladaptive critic behaviors.

In the present strategy, however, the therapist takes the position that "you should *not* stop this behavior right now, but should consider carefully your reasons for doing it, and only then make an informed personal choice about it." This directive often succeeds in getting the client to refrain from self-coercion and thus prevents its detrimental resistive consequences. It also permits the free consideration of the behavior that the client's self-coercion would have preempted.

SOME DYNAMICS OF AMBIVALENCE

To be ambivalent about a behavior is to have reasons for and against engaging in that behavior. From the author's observations, attempting to act totally on one side of one's ambivalence and to disregard the other side seems to heighten the saliency of the reasons on this other side. Consider the commonplace phenomenon of persons who are ambivalent about buying a certain car. Frequently, those individuals who, without ever resolving their ambivalence, disregard their hesitations and just go ahead and buy the car find themselves experiencing "post-buyer's regret." That is, they experience a strong preoccupation with and concern about all of the reasons why they should not have bought the car. In contrast, those who learn that the car they have been considering is about to be sold, and so are being forced to the "don't buy" side, frequently find themselves preoccupied with all of the reasons why they should buy it (see Cialdini's excellent 1993 studies of the influence tactics of sales persons). When one acts on (or is forced to) one side of an ambivalence, one satisfies one's reasons for acting on this side, and these reasons become in a sense "quiescent." However, one leaves unsatisfied the still existing reasons for acting in the opposite way, thus rendering them more salient relative to the satisfied reasons.

In the present strategy, individuals are urged to act temporarily only on one side of their ambivalence when they are urged to continue enacting problematic self-critical behaviors. In doing so, the possibility is created that the reasons to discontinue the behavior, left unsatisfied, gain thereby a greater prominence for the individual.

LOCKING IN CHANGES AND MINIMIZING ANXIETIES ABOUT REGRESSION

Once clients have abandoned their debilitating self-critical ways, they frequently have two reactions, one positive and the other negative. The first of these is that they feel good. This reaction is typified by the following quotes from several persons: "I can't be-

lieve how good I feel"; "These past two weeks have been the best
two weeks of my life"; "I haven't beaten myself up in the last week;
I feel good and I don't think I have anything to work on today."
Among the more common positive changes reported are decreased
depression, enhanced self-esteem, lessened concern with the opinions of others, and greater spontaneous engagement in new and rewarding behaviors that previously were regarded as too risky.

The second, more negative, reaction is that these individuals
often express strong fears that they will not be able to maintain the
gains they have made (Fisch et al., 1982). They fear slipping back
into their old ways. The new way of being and feeling seems to
them very fragile, tentative, and easily lost. The following strategies, all taken or derived from the strategic and solution-oriented
schools of thought (see especially Fisch et al., 1982), have proven
helpful in solidifying clients' senses that they are in control and can
maintain the gains they have made.

PLANNING A RELAPSE

A typical example may convey best the flavor of this strategy.
A client who fears slipping back into old critical ways might be addressed as follows: "You say you are afraid of slipping back. Well,
let me ask you a question which may seem strange. Supposing that
for some reason you actually wanted to go back to your old ways of
criticizing yourself. Can you tell me in detail exactly how you could
do so—how you could deliberately bring this about?" In a manner
reminiscent of the strategy employed with Michael above, clients
are called on to describe, not what might "happen" to "cause" them
to "slip back," but how they could act deliberately to bring this
about. The descriptive language sought from the client is deliberate
action language. "What could you do?" "What would be the next
step you would take?" And so forth. All passive, "happening" language is gently reframed in action language. If the individual reports, for example, "Well, then I think I'd find myself slipping back
into depression," the therapist might counter with, "So, you're fear-
ing a depressive reaction; based on what you've said about your
self-critical actions in the past, what could you do or say to yourself
to produce such a reaction?" In this fashion, clients create for themselves anew a sense that they can control, by their deliberate actions, how they criticize themselves. Frequently, this alone may be
enough to reduce their fears of a relapse. On other occasions, the

therapist might even prescribe a relapse to solidify this sense of personal control (Fisch et al., 1982; Segal, 1991; Weeks & L'Abate, 1982).

SAVING CRITIC ACTS FOR "SPECIAL OCCASIONS"

A good follow-up maneuver, once a deliberate action description has been generated, is to ask individuals if there are circumstances in which they would actually wish to employ their old critical tactics. "The self-critical behaviors you have just described are still in your repertoire," they might be reminded; "Even though you have not been doing them lately, are there any circumstances you can think of for which you would wish to retain them? For example, what if you did something you thought was especially bad, perhaps a serious mistake or morally wrong behavior? Would you want to pull your old self-critical strategies out of mothballs for such occasions to severely punish yourself? Or is there any other circumstance you can think of where you would wish to do so?"

The logic of this inquiry includes a number of elements that are relevant to the matter of clients' senses of control of their self-critical acts. First, the whole line of questioning, consistent with the previous strategy, continues to address the person as one who can elect to employ or not employ the critical actions in question. Second, it reframes those actions, not as the unthinkable, but as overkill sorts of behaviors that the individual may wish to reserve for special occasions. This is designed to get the client away from the classical "Oh, my gosh, whatever I do, I must *not* think of a pink elephant" sorts of dilemmas (cf. Wegner, 1989). The unthinkable is reframed as a thinkable behavioral option that might even be useful in select circumstances. Third and finally, there is an element of subtle encouragement on the part of the therapist to maintain the old self-critical options. The therapist does not join the client in the fearful, "I must not at all costs slip back" way of thinking. In contrast, he or she in a way conveys the message that "this is not some mysterious monster in the closet that will overtake you despite your best efforts—these are behavioral options that you control, and that you may even want to continue to employ, and sensibly so, in certain circumstances."

"PROGRESS IS TWO STEPS FORWARD AND ONE STEP BACK"

Frightening and undermining fears of relapse may also be profitably addressed by reminding persons of the nature of

progress. Too frequently, individuals will encounter one or two negative episodes in which they return to their old critical ways, experience the old depressions and inferiorities, and interpret this a
complete regression (Fisch et al., 1982). In such circumstances, it is
often helpful to remind them that progress is never a relentless onward and upward progression, but rather a "two steps forward,
one step back" sort of affair. The inevitable relapses are reframed,
not as total regressions, but as actual parts of progress. The whole
matter may be taken a bit further by actually stating that you are
suspicious of onward and upward progress. It's too good to be true
and thus not to be trusted, and some backward steps are for this
reason even desirable. The client may be encouraged, if things have
been going exceptionally well, not to go too fast, to make no further
progress, or even perhaps to arrange a relapse on purpose (Fisch et
al., 1982; Segal, 1991).

Using Longer-Term Follow-Up Sessions

One of the elements often involved in fears of regression is
that, after therapy is terminated, individuals will be on their own
should problems develop. One way to minimize such fears is simply to fade sessions out so that the individual has opportunities at
the end of therapy to go for prolonged periods with no therapeutic
assistance. Thus, final sessions might be set at one- or two-month
intervals. In the same vein, the therapist might not officially terminate at all (Segal, 1991), but (his or her circumstances permitting)
merely arrange with clients to discontinue regularly scheduled sessions and to put them on an "as needed" basis. In the author's experience, many clients greet this option with relief. It permits them
to discontinue sessions without feeling that they have irrevocably
shut the door behind them. Most such clients do not in fact return
to therapy. When they do, they tend not to abuse the arrangement
by suddenly calling up and demanding to be seen immediately.

The effectiveness of using prolonged periods may be augment-
ed by homework assignments. For example, a client might be informed that it is almost inevitable that he or she will resort to old
self-critical ways once in a while. Furthermore, the main thing is not
to reduce such occurrences to zero, which is unrealistic, but to be
able to self-correct and recover when they do so. Therefore, as a
homework assignment, they are to watch for and even welcome circumstances where they resort to their old ways, catch themselves
doing so, and work hard to cease what they are doing and employ

other more constructive self-critical measures. Clients are encouraged to make a record of such efforts and to bring these to the following session for discussion.

CONCLUSION

In this chapter, a therapeutic strategy has been described whose primary aim is helping clients to abandon pathological self-critical practices. The central element in this strategy is the employment of a therapeutic prescription to continue destructive self-critical behaviors, but in certain prescribed ways. Theoretical bases, preliminary requirements, follow-up procedures, hypothesized change principles, and some tactics for locking in changes have all been advanced.

Sometimes, the successful implementation of this general strategy is sufficient in itself. The client feels immeasurably better, in control of the old destructive behaviors, and ready to terminate. An important "domino" has been toppled that will lead to further positive changes. At other times, the strategy may be successful, but the indicated course of action is to continue the therapy for awhile and to work on the acquisition of more constructive alternative critic behaviors. At yet other times, the strategy is not successful or it proves impossible to create the initial conditions where it can be employed. All of these scenarios, except the first, necessitate that the therapist possess many more options than this one in his or her therapeutic armamentarium. It is to these other considerations and options that we turn in subsequent chapters.

CHAPTER 6

THE JOB OF THE CRITIC

Criticism is for the benefit of the actor.
                                    PETER G. OSSORIO (1976, p. 172)

Where self-criticism is concerned, doing it right is first a matter of not doing it wrong. When clients cease engaging in their old, self-devastating critical acts, they report very significant changes in how they feel and in how they behave. Self-criticism, however, is a vital and necessary human function. It is at the heart of human self-regulation (Bandura, 1986; Carver & Scheier, 1992; Kanfer, 1971; Meichenbaum, 1973; Ossorio, 1976, 1981, 1990; cf. Vygotsky, 1962). Thus, persons cannot function competently as self-regulating individuals if they cannot perform the job of critic. It is therefore enormously in their interests, not merely to desist from destructive self-criticism, but to become the most competent critics that they are capable of being.

For this reason, a crucial part of psychotherapy for critic problems frequently becomes that of helping clients to acquire positive concepts and skills pertinent to self-criticism. The focus of this chapter will be on the presentation of a number of ideas pertaining to the notion of positive critic function. The focus of the next chapter will be on therapeutic strategies for helping clients to acquire and to utilize such concepts and skills.

PRELIMINARY CONSIDERATIONS

Two-Person Criticism as Heuristic Aid

In general, we are unaccustomed to thinking and talking about the practice of persons constructively criticizing themselves. Further, there is currently very little in the way of theoretical or empirical knowledge available about this matter. In contrast, a great deal more attention has been given to the practice of one person constructively criticizing another. Numerous books and articles have explored, empirically and otherwise, positive approaches to parents criticizing their children (e.g., Hoffman, 1983; McKay, 1992), bosses evaluating their employees (e.g., Ashforth & Cummings, 1983), and teachers appraising the performance of their students (e.g., Paine, Radicchi, Rosellini, Deutchman, & Darch, 1983). In this and ensuing chapters, it will be seen that our knowledge of these two-person situations provides a rich vein of very helpful perspectives for considering the case of persons criticizing themselves (cf. Rehm & Rokke, 1988).

"Criticism Is for the Benefit of the Actor"

This slogan, originally stated by Ossorio (1976, p. 172), captures the positive principle that informs everything else in the present viewpoint. While this entire chapter in some sense will be an elaboration of this principle, let us use two-person situations to begin to capture its basic general point. When we are considering parents with their children, bosses with their employees, teachers with their pupils, or coaches with their players, it is widely understood that the point of criticism ought to be the betterment of the child, the employee, the pupil, or the player. Critics who fail this requirement are almost reflexively criticized: The teacher just assigned a bad grade, but provided no corrective feedback that might help the student to perform better the next time. The boss's criticisms are never focused on what employees are doing right, thus denying them the informational and motivational benefits of such feedback. The parent rebuked the child, but never helped her to understand the moral reasoning behind the rebuke. And so forth. In two-person situations, when criticism does not redound to the benefit of the criticized, it is counted as faulty criticism. Ossorio's essential point is that the same principle applies when the object of criticism is oneself.

The notion of criticism being for the benefit of the actor may be viewed from a second and broader perspective. A dominant and highly respected position holds that persons, if they are to live most fully and meaningfully, would conduct their lives by acting primarily on the basis of their most deeply felt loves, desires, interests, and values. Statements of this position may be found in the work of many prominent authors. For example, the noted anthropologist Joseph Campbell (Campbell & Moyers, 1988) contended that central to the achievement of a full and meaningful life was that one find one's "bliss" and pursue it. By this term, he was referring to those vocational and other paths in life that the individual finds enormously captivating, meaningful, and satisfying. In a similar vein, Carl Rogers (1959) asserted that, in order to live in a way that is fully actualized, persons must act in accordance with their organismic valuing process (i.e., their deepest senses regarding what is intrinsically meaningful and enhancing to them). Finally, the anthropologist Carlos Castaneda (1972), through the utterances of his protagonist, the Indian sage Don Juan, advocated much the same thing when he stated that optimum living inhered in the pursuit of "paths with a heart" (p. 76).

From this perspective, criticism being for the benefit of the actor implies that criticism should serve to help the individual to live in such a fashion. Where it does so, it would be considered beneficial criticism. Where it would fail this test, it would be considered destructive criticism. If Sally loves to play the piano, but as a critic of herself continually berates and degrades herself for any performance less than perfection, she engages in actions that may ultimately lead her either to quit or to hate piano playing. If, on the other hand, she recognizes and works on correcting her errors and weaknesses; acknowledges and appreciates her strengths, her improvements, and the joy of playing itself; and regards perfection as a guide star rather than a standard of adequacy; she stands a far better chance both of becoming a better player and of retaining piano playing as a central joy in her life.

In the present account, then, benefiting the actor stands as the essential criterion for the adequacy of self-critical actions. The hallmark of positive or constructive self-criticism is that it on balance redound to the benefit of the individual. That is, it enables him or her to correct problematic behaviors, to find more successful alternatives, and to recognize and appreciate successful actions. Furthermore, it enables individuals to pursue personally meaningful and fulfilling paths in life. The hallmark of pathological self-criticism is that it on balance damages the individual's ability to behave and, in a wider sense, to participate in life in meaningful and fulfilling ways.

THE JOB OF THE CRITIC

As we learn to walk, to speak a language, to ride a bicycle, to read, to write, to relate to others, or to do anything else of any complexity, we inevitably encounter both successes and failures. As competent socialized adults, we continue to engage in behavior that sometimes proves successful and at other times unsuccessful. This can be seen when we carry on relationships with spouses, children, and friends; when we tackle vocational tasks such as repairing an automobile or treating a client; and when we pursue recreational pastimes such as attending movies or engaging in athletic contests. Clearly, the functioning of persons is very unlike that of highly reliable machines such as lawn mowers and washing machines that for the most part perform correctly every time. It is much more like that of machines such as thermostatically controlled furnaces or chess-playing computers. These devices must monitor conditions, detect when things are within certain desirable boundaries, maintain them when they are within these boundaries, and correct them when they are not (cf. Carver & Scheier, 1992, pp. 502–505 on "negative feedback loops"). We, like them, require both "error detection" and "success detection" capabilities, plus the ability to initiate or not initiate changes, in order to regulate our behavior. In other words, we require critic functions.

From this perspective, it can be seen how self-criticism is a necessary and not (as some authors have alleged) an inherently destructive human function. As thermostatic function is at the heart of furnace regulation, critic function is at the heart of human self-regulation. The central question becomes not whether we should criticize ourselves at all but how we may do so competently and constructively.

OSSORIO'S ANALYSIS OF THE CRITIC'S "JOB"

Ossorio (1976, 1981, 1990) approaches critic function from two perspectives. As an artificial intelligence software designer for the National Aeronautical and Space Administration (NASA), his task is to create self-correcting robotic entities that can adjust to the shifting demands of operating on other planets. As a practicing psychotherapist, his task is to aid persons with problems of self-regulation. Indeed, he has gone so far as to assert that every problem of psychopathology can be formulated as a difficulty with self-regulation (Ossorio, 1976, p. 173; cf. Kanfer, 1970, 1971; Rehm, 1977).

Ossorio (1981, p. 59) has stated that the "job" of the person acting in the role of critic is fourfold: (1) to decide whether things are going satisfactorily, and, if so, (2) to appreciate and enjoy that state of affairs and not to interfere with it. If things are not going satisfactorily, however, the critic's job is (3) to formulate what is going wrong in a way that is usable by the person (diagnosis), and (4) to prescribe ways to make them better (see also Shideler, 1988). The following sections examine each of these four aspects of the job of the critic separately.

TASK 1: TO DECIDE WHETHER THINGS ARE GOING SATISFACTORILY

As critics, our first task is to decide whether things are going satisfactorily. As we monitor the flow of our actions and of our inclinations to act, we also appraise them. Like appraising one's driving, this is often done at a low level of attention, but is brought into sharper focus when the situation requires this. Is the action or temptation okay or not okay? Was it, or will it be, moral or immoral? self-benefiting or self-defeating? appropriate or inappropriate? enjoyable or disagreeable? executed with quality or shabbily done? and so forth for all of the myriad ways in which actions and impulses may be judged okay or not okay.

The appraisals that we render as critics have built-in implications for action (Ossorio, 1990). To say of a completed act that it was okay or not okay in some respect is to say that it should or should not have been done, or should have been done differently. It further implies that, in the future, the act should be repeated, not repeated, or repeated only with modifications. To say of a contemplated act that it is okay or not okay in some respect is to say that this act should or should not be done, or should be done differently.

The Critic as "Screener" of Behaviors

When considering contemplated actions, we are discussing the critic's "screening" function in human self-regulation. In those cases where self-criticism is competently and effectively carried out, a person considers behaviors that he or she has a personal inclination to do and screens out those that are appraised problematic on moral, prudential, hedonic, aesthetic, or other grounds. The set of behaviors that "pass the screen" is comprised of actions that the individual has a personal inclination to do and that are judged nonproblematic. The general result of enacting this set is a life in which a person is for the most part acting on his or her loves, interests, and values in ways that do not create problems (Ossorio, 1976).

The Critic as a Finder of Value

Whatever value a given form of behavior has does not follow from any facts about that behavior (Ossorio, 1976). There are no facts about playing baseball, attending operas, studying psychology, caring for children, or going out on dates that renders them, ipso facto, valuable to all persons. Empirically, what we observe is that some people find each of these activities meaningful and satisfying, while others do not.

As actors or behavers, we give value to forms of behavior. We have places in our lives for all manner of things at various times; e.g., for a new boyfriend or girlfriend, for a vocation, for something that will provide a good evening of entertainment, for a thirst-quenching drink, for a best friend, or for something to give us a sense of purpose in life. As actors (as opposed to critics), we may then give some course of action an opportunity to fill that place in our lives. We may ask Terry out for a date, switch our major to biology, see how that new soft drink serves as a thirst quencher, attend an opera for the first time, or join the Peace Corps. Finally, as critics, we appraise, for better or for worse, how engaging in the behavior that we did filled the place that we asked it to fill. We find Terry (or the new major, or the new soft drink, etc.) satisfying or unsatisfying, or somewhere in between. In other words, while it is up to the actor (the behaving person) to give value, it is up to the critic to accomplish the essential life task of finding value in the going variety of forms of human participation (Ossorio, 1976). (A therapeutic upshot of this analysis might be mentioned briefly. Many clients report that they are unable to find meaning in life. Their characteristic solution attempt is to search for such meaning by scrutinizing as a critic various ways of life. However, the current analysis, as well as the author's clinical experience, suggest that they must first give value by participating in some course of action if they are ever to be able, as a critic, to find such value.)

Pathological Self-Criticism and Task 1

When viewed from the perspective of the first task, the perfectionistic scenarios discussed in Chapter 3 may be seen as especially notable examples of failure at this task. The perfectionist sets standards such that virtually no act or inclination is ever judged satisfactory. No contemplated act is ever good enough, leaving the individual hesitant, doubtful, or even behaviorally paralyzed. No completed act is ever good enough, leaving the individual imbued with a sense of personal failure and often possessed of a feeling that all behavior is ultimately futile.

A second way that persons fail at this task is the diametric opposite of perfectionism. For some critics, anything goes. Too few contemplated actions are found wanting on moral grounds or on grounds that their consequences would be injurious to the larger self-interest of the actor. Thus, little reason is found to refrain from executing these actions promptly and without further ado. Here of course we are touching on the ground of the character disorders— of the psychopath and of other impulsive individuals (Bergner, 1990; Shapiro, 1965).

In both of these scenarios, then, criticism does not redound to the benefit of the actor. Criticism, which ought to serve the self-regulatory functions of screening contemplated courses of action and of evaluating completed ones for future reenactment, fails in these tasks. In these pathological scenarios, the appraisal function has served in the one case to reject everything and in the other to reject nothing.

TASK 2: IF THINGS ARE GOING SATISFACTORILY, APPRECIATE THEM, ENJOY THEM, AND LEAVE THEM ALONE

The second task of the individual operating as a critic has to do with situations in which the actions of the person are found satisfactory. (We will not consider further contemplated actions, because pursuant to the first task, one either enacts or refrains from them.) They are appraised as well done, morally right, personally advantageous, enjoyable, or good in some combination of these and other ways. Here the job of the critic, having recognized this, is to appreciate, to enjoy, and to leave alone (Ossorio, 1981). In its more obvious forms, the person stands back from some completed work—an essay, a discussion with one's child, a room cleaned, an engine tuned—and publicly or privately affirms what has been done:

"Yeah, I like it; I did a good job if I do say so myself." Alternatively, the individual is caught up in some ongoing activity (e.g., pursuing a romantic relationship, working on a project for one's company, or taking a course), recognizes that "this is going well and I'm finding it quite meaningful and absorbing," and then continues to pursue the activity pretty much as before. He or she observes the old maxim that says, "If it ain't broke, don't fix it."

Ossorio's description of this second task is similar in certain of its elements to the practice of self-reinforcement stressed by many cognitive–behavioral theorists and practitioners (e.g., Bandura, 1986; Kanfer, 1970, 1971; Rehm, 1977). Such theorists would consider the individual who privately concludes, "I did a good job if I do say so myself," as a clear-cut instance of self-reinforcement and note that such an action can have three important ramifications. The first of these is motivational. The acknowledgment and appreciation of success in general, whether this comes from others or from oneself, serves as a rewarding state of affairs that is positive in its own right and renders more probable the continuation of such behavior in the future (e.g., Bandura, 1986; Pervin, 1983). The second ramification of such self-reinforcement is informational (Carver & Scheier, 1990): the recognition or understanding derived from the scenario can be that "Behavior X brought me this success (satisfaction, sense of meaning, enjoyment, etc.), and it will probably do so again in the future." The final implication is that such self-reinforcement may enhance the individual's sense of self-efficacy (Bandura, 1977, 1986). The act of appreciating that some course of action has gone well may help individuals to recognize that they possess the competence to behave successfully in particular spheres of their lives. The important consequences of the possession of such self-efficacy beliefs have been amply documented in the research literature (e.g., Cervone, 1989; Schwarzer, 1992).

A Possible Objection

It might be objected at this point that there are times when behaviors are found satisfactory, and yet the person might, quite sensibly, wish to improve the behavior even further. Two points may be made in response to this objection. First, some behavior or course of action might be on balance quite satisfactory but still have its problematic aspects. The relationship is going well generally, but there is some difficulty with openly addressing and resolving issues. The study or work strategy worked fine, but was rather time-consuming. It is generally to these problematic aspects of otherwise quite satisfactory behaviors or courses of action that improvements are addressed. Second, as noted in our earlier discussion of perfectionism, the fact that something can be improved should not be taken as grounds for refusing to appreciate it. The pragmatic upshot of doing so is that, because virtually everything, in principle, can be done better, nothing would ever be appreciated.

Destructive Self-Criticism and Task 2

The primary form of critic failure pertinent to this task is simply failure to appreciate, a phenomenon associated with most of the destructive self-critical patterns discussed in previous chapters. Again, interpersonal situations may serve to bring this notion home in an illuminating way. When the teacher routinely fails to recognize and affirm the good work of the student, when the boss fails to catch the employee getting it right, or when the parent fails to acknowledge and appreciate the right conduct of the child, we recognize that these critics have gone amiss. Further, we recognize the demoralizing effects that such omissions often have on the individuals criticized. As a popular joke puts the matter, "Doing a good job around here is like wetting your pants while wearing a dark suit; it gives you a warm feeling but nobody notices." When persons act well but their actions are never met with recognition, affirmation, appreciation, and even celebration, something is taken away from them. It is much the same when the person whom the critic routinely fails to appreciate is oneself.

TASK 3: IF THINGS ARE NOT GOING SATISFACTORILY,
FORMULATE A USABLE DIAGNOSIS
REGARDING WHAT IS WRONG

Turning to multiperson systems again, we tend easily to recognize descriptions of what is wrong that are not helpful (particularly if we are the recipient of them). During rehearsals, a theater director says to the cast, "No, no, no—that's all wrong; c'mon, we're looking for perfection here." After a botched play, a coach criticizes her player, "Smith, you haven't done a thing right all day; you're useless out there." A parent chastises his child for spilling milk: "Johnny, when are you going to stop being such a klutz?"

In contrast, another director might say, "In that section, you're speaking too rapidly and not conveying a sense that you're absolutely furious at him." Another coach might say, "Smith, you're not staying between your opponent and the goal, that's why you're getting beaten." Another parent might say, "Johnny, you're not picking the cup up by the handle and that's why you're dropping it."

In the first scenarios, the characterizations given of what has gone wrong are of negligible use to the criticized parties. In some cases they are destructive to them. "You didn't do it perfectly . . . you're useless . . . you're a klutz." None of these statements provide any information about what has gone wrong that is usable by the actor to set it right in the future. The last two even suggest to the actor that perhaps he or she is the sort of person who can never get it right. In the second set of scenarios, the opposite is observed. "You're speaking too rapidly"; "You're not staying between your opponent and the goal"; "You're not holding the cup by its handle." All of these convey information about what is going wrong that the actor may assimilate to his or her advantage in correcting the problem.

In criticizing ourselves, the same principle applies. When things have not gone satisfactorily, the job of the critic is to provide descriptions or explanations of what has gone wrong that are usable by the actor (Ossorio, 1981). In some cases, these might be relatively precise diagnoses with clear implications for specific remedial action, such as the examples posed above. In others, they might be as imprecise as "doing it this way doesn't work," which at least tells the actor that, whatever he or she does, it should be something else. The latter leave the option open of generating new and potentially more satisfactory behaviors, not out of logical critic function, but out of one's inclinations or impulses (e.g. "What would feel really good right now?").

Destructive Self-Criticism and Task 3

The self-degradation, hanging judge, and eternal penance scenarios discussed in earlier chapters all entail especially clear failures relative to the third task. In the first of these scenarios, individuals react to perceived failure by turning on themselves and branding themselves with highly undermining, degrading labels. In the second, they attack themselves in a highly vindictive, self-punitive, and unjust fashion. In the third, they engage in endless repetitions of self-flagellating, penitential behavior. In all of these patterns, the self-critical scenario ends with self-denunciatory behavior and its sequelae (depression, low self-esteem, etc.) It does not eventuate in needed behavioral changes, because the sorts of usable diagnoses that persons need to correct actual mistakes, failures, or moral wrongs are not available.

TASK 4: PRESCRIBE WAYS TO IMPROVE MATTERS

The fourth and final task of the critic is to prescribe. That is, based on the sorts of usable diagnoses discussed in connection with the previous task, it is to suggest some alternative behaviors or other modifications that might be implemented to improve problematic states of affairs. Where the director might say "Slow it down" or the coach say "Get between your opponent and the goal," the person acting as self-critic might prescribe to self such things as: "You're getting into one of those mutual silent treatment patterns again with your wife; you'd better get the issue out on the table and try to resolve it as soon as possible"; or "Don't let your time get eaten up again today by all the minutiae; get to the high priority tasks first." Other generally useful prescriptions in certain circumstances might include more open-ended ones such as, "Do what you feel like doing," or "Get out of your rut—do something different." Such prescriptions are useful in situations where one wishes to maximize acting on inclinations and minimize overly tight prescriptions by the critic (e.g., on a Saturday night, a student might wish to get away from his or her study routine and "just do something fun").

Destructive Self-Criticism and Task 4

Where usable diagnoses are lacking, viable prescriptions regarding how to improve matters will be relatively impossible. Thus, the destructive self-critical practices discussed under the third task—self-degradation, hanging judge, and eternal penance—will generally result in failures with respect to the fourth task.

COMPETENT IMPLEMENTATION OF TASKS
AND SELF-REGULATION

In his *Confessions*, the philosopher Augustine lamented that "that which I will, I do not; that which I will not, I do" (1955, p. 135). This may be regarded as a classical expression of a condition of disconnection between critic and actor. As a critic, Augustine is prescribing to himself what he ought and ought not to do, but as an actor he finds himself unable to behave consistently with his own prescriptions. In essence, what he is saying is that he cannot regulate himself. To use our mechanical metaphor, it is as if the thermostat, detecting that the temperature is outside the desired range, is sending "activate" or "deactivate" signals to the furnace, but these are having no influence on the furnace's "behavior."

Self-regulation or self-control implies, then, that there is an operative link between critic and actor. It implies that when persons, operating in the role of critic, screen a contemplated behavior and make the appraisal that it should or should not be done, they are able to follow through with behavior consistent with that appraisal. It implies that, when they make the judgment that some completed behavior should or should not be repeated in the future, they are able to carry out their own prescription with consistent action.

It is the author's clinical observation that, when individuals are able to enact competently the four critic tasks just delineated, they are far more able to regulate their own actions than if they fail to do so by engaging in destructive self-critical actions. A two-person scenario may serve best to explain why this is so. Consider a situation where the regulator and the regulated are two different persons (cf. Rehm & Rokke, 1988); for example, a piano teacher and a pupil. Further, let us consider two different teachers with two different pupils and raise the question as to which of these two teachers is more likely to get her pupil to follow her directions. Teacher 1 recognizes both successful and unsuccessful behaviors, appreciates and at times even celebrates the things her pupil does correctly, corrects the student's mistakes with specific diagnoses, and provides concrete suggestions regarding ways to make things better. Teacher 2, in contrast, imposes humanly impossible standards on her pupil, never notices or appreciates good performance or effort, focuses exclusively on mistakes and failures, and degrades her student with pejorative labels (e.g., "lazy," "untalented"). Furthermore, this teacher attacks the student in excessively punitive ways for mistakes, never lets her forget her bad performances, provides her with no usable feedback regarding her mistakes, and offers no concrete suggestions regarding how matters might be improved. The first teacher is likely to achieve the regulatory end of having her student readily follow her directions. The second teacher creates conditions antithetical to such following. First, there is far less to follow because this teacher has provided no information about successful behaviors, no implementable diagnoses, and no usable prescriptions. Second, the scenario lends itself to reactions such as despair, discouragement, and rebellion, all of which undermine the individual's ability and/or inclination to behave in a manner consistent with the teacher's desires.

SPECIAL CASE: ACTION CRITICIZED IS A DESCRIPTION

Among the actions that persons engage in extensively, and which that are therefore themselves at times the object of self-critical evaluation, are descriptive acts. Persons might say or merely think such things as "I am emotionally alone," "He is into his own world and not really interested in me," "I was rude and thoughtless," "I am not spending enough time with the children," and so on ad infinitum. As can be seen from the examples, some of these descriptions would themselves qualify as self-criticisms (e.g., "I was rude"), while others are intended merely as reports about the way the world is (e.g., "I am emotionally alone").

In multiperson situations, when one person gives a description, others may subject that description to criticism and draw a variety of conclusions. "Yes, I believe what you're saying is well supported by the facts." "Well, I think what you're saying is partially true but . . ." "I really don't think that conclusion follows logically." "That's one way of looking at it, but I think there's a better way." And so on.

One of the jobs of the critic is to subject one's own descriptive acts, critical or otherwise, to the same sort of evaluation as any other action. While doing so with every description would be obsessional and paralyzing, this task becomes important when a specific description has proven problematic (e.g., it has resulted in an individual becoming depressed or engaging in problematic behavior). Is the description okay (consistent with the facts, logical, a helpful view of the matter, etc.)? If so, it may be left to stand. If not, what is wrong with it and how need it be changed so that it becomes an accurate, logical, and functional description?

The clinical importance of this critic function is attested to by the existence of a prominent school of psychotherapy, namely cognitive–behavioral therapy. In this school, the primary focus of attention is on helping persons to criticize and modify their own descriptions when these are found to be problematic (e.g., Beck & Weishaar, 1989; Ellis, 1962; Guidano, 1988; Rehm & Rokke, 1988). As practiced by the highly influential and representative cognitive therapy school (Beck & Emery, 1985; Beck & Weishaar, 1989; Beck et al., 1979), for example, the basic operations involved in this therapy are as follows:

1. Clients who have come to therapy for depression, anxiety, or other difficulties give descriptions of themselves and their worlds.
2. Certain of these descriptions are singled out as highly dysfunctional for the individual (e.g., they result in depression).
3. The therapist and client collaborate in critiquing the adequacy of these descriptions on empirical, logical, and functional grounds.
4. If they are found inadequate in any or all of these ways, attempts are made to eliminate them (e.g., by discerning and altering the underlying schematic beliefs at their root) and to replace them with more adaptive beliefs.

For example, in a widely distributed tape of an actual therapy session, a depressed woman describes herself to Beck as "emotionally alone." She and Beck then evaluate the adequacy of this description on empirical (is it consistent with the facts?), on logical (e.g., is it an overgeneralization?), and on functional (what are the practical consequences of believing it?) grounds. Finding the description problematic on these bases, they conclude together that a different description of the world, one in which the woman is not emotionally alone, is both more accurate and more adaptive.

The desired outcome of cognitive therapy as practiced by Beck and his associates, and one that is representative of other cognitive restructuring approaches, is precisely that persons become more competent and constructive critics of their own descriptions when these prove dysfunctional. It is that they become "their own therapists" in the sense of becoming able to identify, evaluate, and alter such cognitions in the future without benefit of help from a psychotherapist. This goal is entirely consistent with the general thrust of the present book toward helping persons to become competent and constructive critics of themselves. Indeed, it represents an extremely important special case of the wider goals of the present work.

THE CRITIC AS AN ASSIGNER OF STATUS

The film classic *It's a Wonderful Life* provides an excellent example of the point I wish to make in this section. In the film, the protagonist, George Bailey, encounters a crisis in his life when some crucial funds disappear, rendering it likely that his business will become bankrupt and that he will be jailed for embezzlement. George becomes suicidal. Part of what potentiates his suicidal state is that, in George's eyes, this incident represents the latest and worst failure in a history of personal failure. He had always wanted to travel the world, to become educated, to escape his small hometown, and to accomplish great deeds in the wider world. But he has not succeeded in doing any of these. Now, what little he has accomplished, his hand-to-mouth savings and loan company, is going under—a last bitter failure that in his eyes cements his history of failure.

As George is about to jump off a bridge, he is rescued in an interesting way by his guardian angel, Leo. Rather than do the conventional thing and try to talk George out of suicide, Leo jumps into the river himself and calls for help, thus playing upon George's unfailing tendency to give of himself to others. True to form, George saves Leo—and, in the bargain, himself. But his state of mind has not changed and now it is Leo's harder task to get George to alter his suicidal bent. The course of action he ultimately decides on is to try to get George to change his yardstick regarding what constitutes success and failure. He poses a new yardstick, very different from George's current "education, travel, and marvelous deeds" one: "What difference have you made in people's lives?" Summoning his heavenly powers, Leo magically recreates George's community as it would have been had George never been born—an infinitely poorer place where people's lives are far more wretched. After much resistance, George sees the light and accepts Leo's proposed standard of benefiting others. With this acceptance, his own personal history and his world are transformed. It becomes for him "a wonderful life," where even bankruptcy and jail are preferable to death. Fortunately, he is rescued from this fate by the many people whose lives he had so favorably altered.

Critic "Laws"

It is one of the most fundamental choices of adult persons that, as critics, they can set whatever standards or baselines they choose. At some point during his development, George had, as it were, "passed a private law," which decreed that success inhered in such things as becoming educated and going off to the great cities of the world and accomplishing marvelous deeds. This law was written nowhere in stone. In the final analysis, it was George who adopted it and made it binding upon himself. While many in the American culture then and now would endorse such a standard for success, many others would not, including George's family and many friends who already found him a good and even great man.

Not only did George pass this law, but also, in light of his transgression of it, declared himself a failure. It was he who was responsible ultimately for assigning to himself this status in the world. When Leo came on the scene, he (not unlike our "reframing" colleagues) took it as his principal task to present a new critic standard to George—success as inhering in making a contribution to the betterment of people's lives—and persuade him to adopt it. George's ultimate adoption of this new critic standard radically transformed his self-assigned place or status in the world from that of failure to that of success, now reformulated as contributor to a better world.

As critics, we pass laws and, based on our appraisal of our own fulfillment or transgression of these, assign to ourselves various places in the world. Though a cinematic and fictional one, the above example captures the enormous difference—at times a life and death difference—that our fulfillment of these laws can make. As critics we may pass and uphold laws that are reasonable and viable for ourselves, or we may fail to do so. We may declare ourselves successes or failures, somethings or nothings, good or evil persons, caring or selfish individuals, all depending on the standards we create and uphold.

SELF-STATUS ASSIGNMENT AND REALISM

In concluding this section, a note about realism is in order. It may seem from what has been said here that one's status is entirely a matter of what one declares it to be, based on whatever standards one elects to uphold. This is not a correct surmise. Consideration of a simpler matter will perhaps best capture the present position. Suppose there is in front of me a rock. The limits of what I can take this rock to be—the limits of what places I can assign it in my world—correspond to the limits of what I can successfully treat it as being. Thus I may realistically regard it as a paperweight, a weapon, an object that obeys Newton's laws, a container of a geologic record, and more. I may not realistically regard it as a calculator, a hair dryer, or a book because I cannot carry off such claims by doing calculations, drying my hair, or reading it. In the same way, the limits on what we can appraise ourselves as being are considerable but not infinite and (barring delusion) not totally the product of our own decisions. George Bailey may not regard himself realistically as the wealthiest, the most diplomatic, or the best-educated person in town, but he may regard himself as someone whose contribution to the lives of many others has been invaluable. The bounds of the realistic are considerable. Again, they are so considerable that the happiness of persons and even their life or death can depend on how they exercise critic functions within them.

CONCLUSION

In this chapter, a description of positive critic function has been presented. Following the work of Ossorio, the perspective adopted has been that self-criticism is for the benefit of the actor. That is, its ultimate purpose, and the ultimate criterion of its adequacy, should be the improvement of an individual's behavior and, ultimately, improvement in the quality of his or her participation in life. It was further demonstrated that self-criticism is not an unfortunate, inherently pathological human function, but an activity that is utterly central to human self-regulation. The fourfold job of the critic in this self-regulatory process was described at some length. Finally, the awesome power of the critic as a "passer of laws" and an assigner of statuses, and the consequent necessity that persons pass viable laws for themselves, was described.

In the following chapter, the focus of attention will shift to therapeutic strategies for helping persons to adopt the more constructive, beneficial approaches to self-criticism that have been described above.

CHAPTER 7

PROMOTING CONSTRUCTIVE MODES OF SELF-CRITICISM

It is easiest to give up an invalid approach when one has a
more effective alternative to try instead.
RICHARD DRISCOLL (1984, p. 167)

In this chapter, the focus of attention will shift to therapeutic interventions designed to enable clients to learn and to implement constructive self-critical behaviors. Topics discussed will include (1) the
use of therapeutic images and concepts as means for conveying important ideas about the form that such alternative behaviors might
take; and (2) the employment of various behavioral directives and
other procedures to help individuals to engage actively in such behaviors. The general understanding here, as throughout this book,
is that no single approach will be possible or most effective with all
clients. Thus, the attempt is to provide the therapist with options
that may be used with different clients who prove amenable to different interventions.

In accomplishing the goals described in this chapter, it has
proven extremely helpful to heed the advice of Milton Erickson that
in psychotherapy one does well to "utilize" and build on what is already there (Erickson, 1985; O'Hanlon, 1987). Thus, in promoting
constructive self-critical perspectives and practices with clients, the
more that we can build on their existing values, motivations, under-

standings, competencies, and world views—and, conversely, the less that we can come into conflict with these—the better clients will be able to hear, understand, and use what is presented.

THE USE OF IMAGES

Virtually anything pertinent to competent critic function may be conveyed to clients through the use of social role images such as those of parent, boss, teacher, coach, or pastor. The primary reason for employment of such images is that most clients with critic problems lack a concept of constructive self-criticism, but do possess valuable concepts and understandings pertaining to how persons in such roles would constructively criticize others in their charge.

By way of illustration, a therapist might be interested in conveying the perspective contained in the earlier quote, "Criticism is for the benefit of the actor." As noted in the previous chapter, this aphorism expresses the perspective on self-criticism that its reason for being should be to enhance the quality of the behavior, and thus the quality of life, of the person criticized. While few clients will exhibit a command of this perspective in the case of self-criticism, almost all will understand it in the case of one person criticizing another. Thus, the latter understanding becomes an excellent vehicle to communicate the perspective. For example, almost all clients easily recognize that if a dance instructor criticizes by degrading ("You clumsy oaf; you'll never get it right"), this is bad criticism because it disqualifies the dancer and renders him or her less able, not more able, to dance. In contrast, they recognize that a dance instructor who appreciates it when things go right ("Yes! That's it. Well done!") and who corrects with constructive, implementable prescriptions when things go wrong ("Not that way, Terry. Now watch me. Turn your foot this way") is doing a good job as a critic precisely because such criticism is likely to benefit the performance of the dancer.

SELECTING THE BEST IMAGES
FOR SPECIFIC CLIENTS

In selecting a social role image for use with a specific client, three criteria should be kept in mind. All are special cases of observing the Ericksonian policy of building on persons' existing knowledge, values, competencies, interests, and other personal characteristics. First, the client should possess a good understanding of the role captured by the image and, most importantly, a good understanding of what competent and constructive enactment of that role would look like. If he or she does not have a sufficient grasp of these matters, the therapist's illustrations and appeals may serve only to leave the client bewildered. Thus, for example, many persons with critic problems have had parents who fulfilled their parental roles in rather poor and problematic ways. Some of these clients will not understand therapist appeals to what normative or good parents do, and will find the use of this image unhelpful (and even aversive).

The second criterion when selecting a social role image is that the individual should value that role and the whole way of behaving that it captures. The person, for example, who values what good coaches do for their athletes will appreciate the worth that inheres in constructively fulfilling the critic functions that are part of that role. In contrast, the individual who thinks that athletic activities are stupid and meaningless and that all coaches are abusive tyrants will find little of merit in illustrations that appeal to this image.

The third and final criterion for image selection is that clients should show some resonance to its use. In the language of the hypnotists, the therapist should look for "responsiveness" when he or she is using the image. Does the image at least hold the client's interest? More desirably, does it "grab" or captivate him or her? If the image does not accomplish at least the former, it should be abandoned.

If all three of these conditions are met, the therapist is in a position to capitalize on a highly valuable resource possessed by the client. The latter has a social role concept (e.g., that of parent) that codifies a complex perspective and way of behaving. Further, he or she finds the relationship and attendant way of behaving a valuable and meaningful one—and an intriguing one when introduced as a model for how to criticize oneself. There is here a "package," as it were, of understandings, perspectives, values, and skills that the therapist can assimilate to the enormous benefit of the client. The therapist is not attempting the difficult task of creating something from nothing. Rather, he or she is taking an already existing resource from one area of the client's life and attempting to bring it to bear in another area, self-criticism.

"Parent"

Perhaps the most generally useful social role image is that of "parent." As employed here, the term refers not to the mere fact of biological antecedence, but to the relational role implied by this term. What is central to this role is parental love—a personal care for and commitment to the best interests of one's child, understood as a commitment to doing one's best to enable that child to become a competent, socialized, moral, meaningfully participating adult (Hardison, 1991). In this culture, as in most, it is generally understood that this larger good will be brought about by the undertaking of certain specific tasks. These include those of nurturing, guiding, protecting, disciplining, and supporting one's child (Hardison, 1991).

Persons are evaluated as "doing a good job as a parent," then, to the degree that they are both (1) committed to the larger goal of acting in the best interests of their children, and (2) competently undertaking the specific jobs or tasks that comprise the parental role. When persons exhibit caring and commitment to their children but cannot discharge parental tasks competently, they are judged to be "loving well but not wisely." When they exercise behavioral competencies adequately but lack a true investment in their children's welfare, they are seen as "going through the motions"; as doing all the things that parents are supposed to do but without the motivation that ideally would infuse the effort (Hardison, 1991). The present conception is consistent with Baumrind's (1967, 1983) findings that it is the combination of optimum parental behaviors and an optimum relationship that is most conducive to a host of positive developmental outcomes (see also Kuczynski, Zahn-Waxler, & Radke-Yarrow, 1987; Maccoby & Martin, 1983).

Permeating the various tasks of parenthood such as guidance, discipline, and support is the need for parents to function as critics of their children. In this role of critic, their first major job centers around recognizing and appreciating what is positive and functional in their children (Hardison, 1991). It is that of noticing, accepting, and affirming those behaviors, accomplishments, traits, interests, and abilities of their children that are positive (e.g., the child's friendliness, love of drawing, or efforts in an athletic event). The second major job of parents as critics is that of identifying and of attempting to help their children to alter behaviors and characteristics that are problematic (e.g., excessive aggressiveness or a tendency to give up too easily in the face of difficult tasks) (Hardison, 1991; Hoffman, 1988).

Using the Parent Concept Therapeutically

Employing this perspective of a parent/critic with clients who possess and value it, numerous therapeutic options are possible. A number of these will be mentioned later in this chapter in other connections. Here, only one will be noted. Clients might be asked to view a wide variety of destructive things that they do to themselves through the perspective of a parent criticizing his or her child. With their own (actual or hypothetical) child, would they systematically focus on negatives and never appreciate positives? crucify their children for anything less than perfection? never acknowledge that anything their children did was successful? brand them with disqualifying labels? If their children were attacked by hostile critics, would they join the chorus of the critics as they do in their own case? What do they believe the consequences would be if they did employ any of the above measures? What alternative critical approaches would they employ with their children to correct problematic behaviors and why would they do so?

For example, during a session, a client might report that she made what she considers to be a serious error the past week, and that she has been attacking herself vigorously for it. If the image of "parent" has been introduced, and the client has exhibited some understanding, competency, and value for that relational role, the therapist might suggest: "I'd like you to come over here to this chair and try to picture if you can that it's your daughter, not you, who has made that mistake and is sitting in that other, empty chair. Now, you believe it really is a serious mistake. You don't want to let it slide. You want to help her to correct it. Why don't you speak to her as a mother. What would you say to her to deal with this matter?" If the therapist has been correct in his or her initial assessment that the client knew how to function as a good parental critic, the client typically will correct the child without resorting to degradation, viciousness, or the imposition of impossible standards. Corrective feedback and suggestions may be supplied by the therapist if the individual struggles with this task. This mode of critical reaction then can be posed as a possible approach to herself, any resistances to implementing it can be addressed (see Chapter 8), and an agreement may be reached that the client will attempt to respond to two mistakes in the following week in this more constructive manner. Such homework should always be reviewed in the following session in order to assess the client's cooperation, to determine the effectiveness of doing the assignment, to provide feedback, and to acknowledge and appreciate the client's efforts.

What one observes when one poses such questions of well-chosen clients is that it calls on them to adopt a different, far more constructive perspective on self-criticism. Using the resource of their knowledge, skills, and values for competent parenting, they are able to distinguish more clearly what is constructive and what is destructive. Further, they can appraise better the consequences of various courses of action and can devise new, more beneficial solutions for themselves. Finally, because parents are partly in the business of correcting mistakes and weaknesses, they can see that using this approach is not an ultrapermissive, "anything goes" sort of affair, which for many persons would be grounds for dismissing it.

Using Relational Aspects of Parent Concept

The above measures largely concern the employment of procedural or behavioral competencies from one sphere of life in the service of promoting positive change in another. "How would you behave and not behave with your children," the logic goes, "and can you see how the same considerations would extend to the treatment of yourself?" Beyond this, however, are the less procedural, more relational elements inherent in the parental role that, as noted above, are centrally concerned with a commitment to act in the best interests of one's child. These elements, too, comprise something with considerable transfer value.

It is possible to have a relationship with oneself that has as its core element a commitment to act in one's own best interests. In this context, this is understood not as a narcissistic, "me first," agenda, but as a commitment that takes its basic form from the commitment of parent to child. "To act in your best interests" thus becomes a commitment to doing one's best to enable oneself to be a competent, moral, fulfilled, participating individual. Expressed negatively, it becomes a commitment to refuse to engage in forms of criticism that are abusive and destructive such as self-degradation, perfectionism, and harsh self-punitiveness.

Essentially, this parental commitment can be proposed straightforwardly to clients as an alternative to their current self-abusive agendas. The parental agenda takes the essential form: "My job is to take care of you by acting in your best interests." Clients' current ones frequently take forms such as, "My job is to rub your face in the ugly truth," "not give you any sort of approval until you shape up," "never to let you feel good about yourself lest you become conceited," or "to dangle the carrot of approval always a little beyond you to keep you motivated." In general, it is helpful to contrast the two perspectives explicitly for clients. They may then be asked to consider carefully which of them would be most likely to help their children to lead meaningful, responsible, participatory lives and which would most likely help them to do so. If they decide that the agenda to act in their own best interests is the better one, they may be encouraged in the direction of making a personal commitment to treat themselves in this fashion (Rubin, 1975).

The many popular books, some of them quite good (e.g., Stone & Stone, 1993), that advocate the desirability of "parenting" oneself in positive ways seem to be making a point similar to this one. However, too often they neglect the fact that constructive negative criticism and discipline are essential parts of the parental role. What emerges is a portrait of parenting oneself that comes across as indulging oneself.

Conclusion

In these and other ways, the image of a parent who is acting competently and caringly in the best interests of a child, which selected clients already possess, may become the model for something they do not possess: the concept of a competent, caring self-critic.

"Boss"

In much the same way as that described for the image of a parent, the concepts of the teacher, boss, coach, arts instructor, clergyman, etc., who is dedicated to the best interests of those in his or her care may be employed. Because the general logic of the employment of all of these images is essentially identical to that described for the parental one, only one additional image, that of "boss," will be discussed.

The destructive critics who tend to benefit most from the boss image are perfectionistic individuals who drive themselves harshly and relentlessly for achievement and productivity (see Bergner's 1981 portrait of the obsessive-compulsive individual as an "overseer" to self). These individuals are analogous to bosses who are harsh and punitive, relentlessly coercive, never satisfied with their employees' efforts, exclusively focused on imperfections as opposed to successes, and disregarding of their employee's feelings and interests. While such persons are effective to some extent, they also engender enormous resistance, abysmal morale, and even rebellion (e.g., work slowdowns, absences, and strikes). The upshot of all of this is a reduction in the productivity the boss so much desires.

When one examines the literature on leadership in management contexts (e.g., Bennis, 1989; DePree, 1989), the picture that emerges of effective leaders includes a number of characteristics. For example, effective leaders typically (1) set high but reachable standards; (2) give explicit recognition for worker efforts and accomplishments; (3) consider their employees' ideas, needs, and feelings; and (4) employ modes of correction that are firm and clear without being overly punitive or degrading. Leaders who conduct themselves in such fashions are typically a great deal more effective than their "overseer" counterparts in enlisting the cooperative efforts of those under their authority and in achieving outcomes marked by excellence.

As in the case of the parent image, the author has found it profitable first to introduce the concept of such a competent boss or leader to carefully selected individuals. Again, care is taken to emphasize its compatibility with their existing values (in these cases, productivity, achievement, and excellence tend to be quite important). Then, when appropriate situations arise, relevant questions utilizing the client's command of this boss perspective may be employed. For example, with one client, Sheila, who was known as a rather effective and supportive supervisor in her agency, the following questions were posed and pursued: "Would you drive your supervisees relentlessly from morning to night the way that you do yourself? Would you pressure them to make every minute productive, and accuse them of "laziness" and "irresponsibility" if they took the least little break or wanted a night out with their families? How would you expect them to respond if you did so? Would you expect more productivity or better quality work? How do you in fact approach them and how does it work out?" With Sheila, it proved possible, after some initial resistance, to bring the excellent judgment and human qualities she brought to her work as a supervisor into the service of "supervising" herself in a far more benign and effective manner.

THE "NASTY THERMOSTAT"

Some highly self-critical clients cannot benefit from the employment of social role concepts such as "parent," "teacher," "boss," or "friend." While they might possess them in a rudimentary way, their relational lives have been so impoverished or aversive that they do not know in any full sense what a friend or a parent is, and are often quite cynical about such notions. For such persons, one option that the therapist can employ is that of using images and metaphors from the world of mechanical systems. One of the author's favorites is the somewhat whimsical image of "the nasty thermostat."

Larry, a computer programmer for a large national organization, had had an extremely painful childhood and adolescence in which he had been the target of a great deal of humiliating criticism and ostracism from his family and peers. This personal history had resulted in a poor understanding of other persons and a harsh, cynical outlook on them. It had also resulted in him being an absolutely scathing, hateful critic of himself. Somehow, however, he had retained a rather good sense of humor. When the ill-considered attempt to use a parental metaphor with Larry met with a hostile and cynical reaction and also revealed a radical ignorance on his part of how good parents behaved, it was dropped immediately. Given his mastery of nonpersonal systems and his sense of humor, however, the following general line was taken with Larry to try to convey the basic problem with how he criticized himself: "Think of your home heating system. Part of that system of course is your thermostat, and it has certain jobs to do. Basically, when the temperature in your house is within a certain desirable range, its job is to recognize this state of affairs and leave well enough alone; its job is to do nothing. However, when it gets too cold or too hot, its job is to recognize that things are outside the desirable range and to do something about it—to turn the furnace on or turn it off. When it's working as it's supposed to be working, that's what it does. Now think about a thermostat that does something quite different. When it detects that the house has gotten too hot, it just yells down to the furnace: "You are a really crappy furnace," and goes on to berate the furnace roundly. It doesn't do anything else, such as turn the furnace off—it just puts it down. Well, in a way, that's what you're doing. The whole point of you functioning as a critic is to recognize when things are going right and to leave them alone, and to recognize when they are going wrong and to figure out what's wrong and do something to correct yourself. But instead, it looks like you get stuck attacking yourself, and that gets in the way of correcting yourself. You are like that nasty thermostat." In Larry's case, the idea of a furnace calling down epithets upon itself proved an amusingly ridiculous one and he got the point. Subsequent to this, the metaphor was used again in other contexts (e.g., a "perfectionistic thermostat" that berated itself for turning the furnace off at 70.1023 degrees rather than at 70.0000 degrees), and became a shared joke/image between therapist and client.

THE USE OF CONCEPTS

In addition to the use of images, a second means for helping clients to achieve important understandings and perspectives on self-criticism is that of educating them about relevant concepts. Just as many cognitive-behavioral therapists (e.g., Lange & Jakubowski, 1976) take great pains to convey to their clients the concept of "assertion" (vs. "aggression"), so the therapist here may resort to the educational task of seeing to it that clients acquire useful concepts pertaining to self-criticism. Three such concepts will be discussed in this section, those of charity, forgiveness, and compassion.

CHARITY

Charity has been defined by Webster as "forbearance in judging others; leniency" (1985, p. 250). A more practically implementable definition, for the psychotherapist's purposes, is the notion that charity is "an exploitation of the least invidious yet realistic conceptual possibilities" (Ossorio, personal communication, 1972). It is the choice, given two or more applicable descriptions of the same thing, of the least invidious of these (cf. the popular notion of "giving the benefit of the doubt"). When seen in this light, charity can be framed usefully as a cognitive policy wherein, given a choice between two realistic ways of interpreting one's own actions or characteristics, one systematically chooses the least destructive of the two.

To illustrate this concept in a way that the author sometimes does with clients, let us suppose that the wife of an individual is given to spending a good deal of time attending to her personal appearance. The husband might, with roughly equal realism, construe her behavior in a variety of quite disparate ways. He might see his wife as "vain" or "overly concerned with external appearances," and thus a rightful object of his scorn. Or he might take it that she is "feminine," that this is "just her way," and/or that her behavior arises out of a very human and understandable insecurity but is in no sense contemptible. These characterizations of her actions may not differ in realism. They do, however, differ in charity as defined above and, because of this, in their consequences. Depending on the appraisal chosen, the wife may be seen and treated as anything from an object of contempt to a normal, understandable person for whom it is important to look good. All of these considerations apply, point for point, when the object of criticism is oneself.

Destructively self-critical individuals tend to select more uncharitable, destructive interpretations of events in their relations with themselves. The imparting and clarification of the concept of charity, coupled with an encouragement to adopt and practice such charity in a systematic way (see the following section on the promotion of alternative critic activities), has proven a helpful approach with these self-critical persons. In particular, it has proven useful with the individuals discussed above whose relational histories have been so impoverished or aversive that they lack an understanding of positive human roles and relationships. Such persons do far better with more concrete policy concepts that do not presuppose much in the way of the possession of such relational understandings. Finally, some clients, particularly those who are quite cynical and antagonistic toward anything they deem sentimental, will respond negatively to the word "charity." With such persons, a different locution should be adopted that seems more likely to gain acceptance. These might include "functional alternativism," "adaptive reframing," "or cognitive restructuring," all of which have a more scientific, less humanistic ring to them.

FORGIVENESS

Many pathologically self-critical persons, and especially those involved in the "eternal penance" scenario described earlier, are badly in need of self-forgiveness. However, when it is suggested by a well-meaning friend or loved one that they should "forgive themselves," they are genuinely and understandably at a loss as to how to go about doing so. With this in mind, the concept of forgiveness, like that of charity, will be formulated here in such a way that it heuristically suggests concrete behaviors that might be undertaken to accomplish it. In the language of psychological research, we are here defining the term in such a way as to permit more readily its operationalization.

To forgive in the fullest possible sense is to restore the accused to full community standing (Camden, 1993). It is to come to a personal position toward the accused in which he or she is no longer hated or resented, is no longer regarded as in need of making further reparation for his or her transgression (cf. "forgiving a debt"), and is no longer rejected, ostracized, or given a diminished community standing. Thus, for example, a woman who had completely forgiven her husband for a marital infidelity would be one who had ceased to be angry or hateful toward him for his transgression, had stopped feeling that he needed to "make it up to her" any further, and had included him fully in her life again as a husband. Of course, in most actual cases, forgiveness might be present to a considerable degree, but not be so complete as this. For example, the woman in our example might no longer be resentful toward her husband or feel that he needed to make further reparations, but might have decided to proceed slowly in the matter of including him again in her life as a full and trusted partner.

The behavioral implications of this definition become evident when we recognize that forgiveness rests on a critic appraisal. The wife in our example cannot, after her husband's transgression, simply decide to turn off her anger, her feeling of being betrayed, or her strong reluctance to reinstate him as a trusted husband. To accomplish such things—to forgive him—she must see the world in such a way as to call for them. She must appraise matters in such a way that these acts of forgiveness make genuine sense to her. For example, suppose that what she observes in the year after the infidelity is that her husband confesses his guilt, acknowledges his responsibility for wrongdoing, and expresses a strong and genuine remorse. Furthermore, he vows that he will never again be unfaithful and backs all of this up with actions over a significant period of time that are consistent with his verbal avowals. Observing all of this, his wife might come to the following view: "He is genuinely sorry. His infidelity was not an expression of the sort of person he is or of the love or commitment he has toward me, but is an aberration. He has gone to the ends of the earth to make it up to me and show me how sorry he is. Overall, it looks to me like he does love me, is committed to our relationship, and is resolved never to do this sort of thing again." In the wake of such a critic appraisal, the wife may be able genuinely to forgive her husband.

All of the considerations contained in Camden's general formulation of forgiveness apply point for point when the individual whom one cannot forgive is oneself. And, because forgiveness follows from the rendering of certain critic appraisals, the tasks of therapy in these cases are to raise the sorts of questions and to engage in the sorts of dialogue that will enable clients to come to such forgiveness-generating appraisals.

Depending on the specific client, the kinds of questions that might be raised to achieve such appraisals include the following: Are there in fact transgressions of a significant nature? (In cases where there are not, correction of the client's misconception may constitute the exclusive focus of discussion.) Is the client regretful or remorseful for the transgression(s) (a tendentious question to pose of these unforgiving clients, but one still worth raising since it elicits public confessional behavior that may be helpful)? Is the client committed to refraining from the transgressive behavior in the future? Has he or she already refrained, perhaps for prolonged periods of time? Was the behavior in character or out of character for the person, or was it an aberration (the realization that a transgression represented an aberrant action not in keeping with one's character can be very powerful)? Were there mitigating circumstances that the client has ignored in his or her appraisal of self? Has the client suffered enough or made sufficient restitution in light of the severity of the transgression?

In raising and discussing such matters, the device of exploiting the client's judgmental competence with regard to interpersonal situations may again be employed profitably. For example, some of the above questions might be raised in the following manner. "If you were a judge in the legal system, would you say that the statute of limitations had expired in this case?" "If your best friend, _____, had done this, would you accuse and punish her again and again for the same 'crime,' tens and even hundreds of times over years and years? When would you say she has 'suffered enough' or 'paid the price' enough?"

The above questions are not posed with an assumption that the answers will always be easy ones for clients. Some persons who cannot forgive themselves have done things such as abused alcohol for years and neglected their families, mistreated their children and spouses physically or emotionally, destroyed a relationship through their uncaring treatment of another, or other similarly objectionable things. They may decide, quite reasonably, that there remains a need for them to make a serious commitment to changing their behavior over a prolonged period of time, or that further restitution is in order, or that some other pertinent course of action is needed before they can make the appraisals requisite for self-forgiveness. Such persons will not be satisfied with easy reassurances from the therapist that they need not do so. In such cases, it should be noted that, while self-forgiveness cannot be easy or quick, voluntarily and sincerely stating one's remorse and undertaking some manner of signicant reparational action brings with it for many people a considerable measure of self-forgiveness. Even if they are not yet "redeemed" (understood in a secular sense here), they feel immeasurably better about themselves for embarking on "the road to redemption."

There is a final element that therapists would do well to bear in mind in connection with self-forgiveness. As noted in Chapter 3, there are explicit ceremonies or rituals of atonement that are institutionalized in our culture and that most persons understand (at least implicitly). Religious rituals of confession are perhaps the clearest instance of these. In such rituals, when all goes according to plan, the transgressor pursues forgiveness from another, and through this medium achieves self-forgiveness. In a therapeutic context, self-unforgiving clients are engaging in behavior that is similar in many respects to persons in atonement ceremonies. They are, for example, reporting their transgressions, expressing their remorse, and relating how they have "flogged" themselves innumerable times for their offense, to another human being. If the latter individual, the therapist, is able to listen to these reports and respond in a manner that is genuinely accepting of the individual, this will function often much in the manner of the external forgiveness that is offered in ritualized atonement ceremonies such as religious confession. Thus, the sort of acceptance that was originally promoted by Rogers (1951) and has since been adopted by therapists of many schools (e.g., Beck & Weishaar, 1989; Kohut, 1977; Wilson, 1989) can be immeasurably helpful in achieving the therapeutic goal of self-forgiveness.

COMPASSION

The concept of compassion was originally introduced by the psychoanalyst Rubin (1975) in his important work on self-hatred. It was subsequently adopted and strongly emphasized in the cognitive–behavioral approach to self-criticism of McKay and Fanning (1992). The latter authors attempted in their work to formulate Rubin's somewhat unsystematic comments on this topic into a tighter conceptualization that would suggest actual behavioral operations that their clients could implement. They stated that compassion could be considered a skill having three distinct components: understanding, acceptance, and forgiveness. Let us consider their treatment of each of these in turn.

By understanding, McKay and Fanning are referring to an insightful comprehension of the source of one's own problems that is framed in sympathetic, supportive, nondegrading terms (1992, p. 84). This definition is similar to the everyday use of the term as in the sentence, "She proved to be very understanding about my problems." Here, individuals strive, as a matter of policy, to seek insights and explanations of their difficulties that are more benign and sympathetic, as opposed to self-hating. McKay and Fanning relate the example of Sean, a brick mason, who was under extremely heavy pressure at work and one evening found himself contemplating binging on snack foods in front of the television. In contrast to his usual reaction to such behavior, which was angrily self-contemptuous, Sean had the sudden realization that such binging was a very human and understandable way he had of consoling himself after days when he was extremely stressed. This explanation permitted him a useful insight into the problem, and one that did not result in his customary habit of heaping abuse on himself.

Acceptance, according to McKay and Fanning, is an "acknowledgment of the facts, with all value judgments suspended" (1992, p. 85). In this regard, the achievement they strive for with their clients is one in which the latter can look squarely at certain less fortunate facts about themselves, acknowledge them as facts, and refuse to use them as ammunition for self-hating attacks. For example, persons might look at such things as their physical unattractiveness, their shyness, their lack of assertiveness, or some other unfortunate characteristic, and strive to adopt an attitude that, "This is a fact about me; I may not like it; I may wish that I were better looking (more assertive, less shy, etc); but I steadfastly refuse to use this as ammunition to abuse and reject myself."

By forgiveness, McKay and Fanning are referring to the achievement of what they term a "case closed" (1992, p. 86) attitude toward their own past mistakes, failures, and transgressions. It is essentially a refusal to attack oneself over and over again for the same "crime." Expressed positively, it is a letting go of the old crime and of any intentions to prosecute further, to seek revengeful self-punishment, or to exact future reparation or restitution. In a manner somewhat similar to what was said previously in this section,

McKay and Fanning assert that such self-forgiveness "flows out of understanding and acceptance" (1992, p. 86).

In their respective therapies, Rubin, as well as McKay and Fanning, engage in explicit didactic work elucidating the concept of compassion and its various components. Further, they exhort their clients to practice actively such compassionate modes of responding to their own mistakes, failures, and moral transgressions. Of the two approaches, the latter, cognitive–behavioral one, has placed a greater emphasis on operationalizing compassionate responses in ways that clients can engage in them more readily.

URGING THE CLIENT TO PRACTICE CONSTRUCTIVE SELF-CRITICISM

Once clients have recognized clearly that they are the perpetrators of destructive self-critical behaviors and have shown some acceptance of the idea that alternative critic behaviors may do a more effective and less costly job of accomplishing their personal objectives, it is important that they be engaged actively in these alternative behaviors. Such active engagement is imperative for a number of reasons.

First and most basically, success in the present therapeutic approach resides in persons actively treating themselves in new, more constructive ways. Merely talking about the constructive alternatives captured above in the images, concepts, or critic "job description" will not suffice. Clients' current problems lie in how they are behaving as critics toward themselves, and the solution to these problems lies in their behaving differently.

Second, the goal of behavioral change does not imply merely that clients engage in different performances, but also that their actions become true expressions of the relationship they have to themselves. (Compare: If we were attempting to help a mother alter destructive behaviors toward her child, we would not be satisfied with an outcome where the mother changed to more constructive behaviors but continued to dislike the child.) To achieve such an outcome, one of the things we would do well to set in motion is the relationship change formula: "If the behavior of X vis-à-vis Y is *not* an expression of the relationship which holds between them (namely, R), then that relationship will tend to change in the direction of one for which the behavior that *did* occur *would* have been an expression" (Ossorio, 1981, p. 71; emphases in original). Thus, just as when I invite a new colleague over for dinner my relationship with that person will tend to change from one of being strangers to one of being friends, so when I begin to treat myself in more caring ways my relationship with myself will tend to change toward a more self-liking one. To set this relationship change process in motion, it is important that clients begin during therapy to behave differently toward themselves.

A third reason for promoting active engagement in new critic behaviors is that, in the course of learning to criticize themselves differently, clients will almost inevitably encounter resistances, mistakes, and difficulties (see the next chapter). Thus, if they are engaging actively in trying out these new modes of self-criticism as therapy proceeds, the therapist can be available as a valuable resource to help them to overcome these obstacles.

Fourth and finally, active practice in the specific form of homework is a desirable element in this as in other psychotherapies (e.g., Beck & Weishaar, 1989; DeShazer, 1988; Driscoll, 1984; Segal, 1991). When it is employed, therapy is not confined to the hour, but extends throughout the week. It is not a passively received treatment, but a process in which clients become active coparticipants. The contrast between persons who have been working actively on their own behalfs all week and clients who come in saying, "I can't remember what we talked about last week," could not be more stark. Nor could the differences, other things being equal, between the rates at which these clients will improve.

For all of these reasons, then, the focus in this section will be on relating some therapeutic means for helping clients to become actively involved in criticizing themselves differently. The following recommendations will include some procedures that may be implemented within the therapy hour and others that may be employed as homework assignments.

COLLABORATIVE NEGOTIATION OF CRITIC APPRAISALS

Collaborative negotiation of critic appraisals between therapists and clients is one primary method of helping the latter to practice alternative critic behaviors. This procedure is similar to that employed by Beck and his associates (Beck & Emery, 1985; Beck & Weishaar, 1989; Beck et al., 1979) in their well-known technique of collaborative empiricism. The present approach, however, places a somewhat greater emphasis on the form (vs. the content) of the self-critical behavior.

In collaborative negotiation, the client presents, often in the course of merely relating his or her problems, a self-appraisal that seems highly maladaptive (e.g., a self-degrading one to the effect that "I am unlovable"). The therapist, discerning the destructive character of this appraisal, singles it out for the client's attention. The two of them might discuss conjointly the consequences of this self-degradation. For example, its attribution of a highly disqualifying insufficiency makes it grounds for such emotions as despair and sadness, for a state of demotivation, for inactivity in the romantic arena, and for foregoing any sort of useful investigation of how one's romantic difficulties might be remedied.

Having jointly recognized the deleterious consequences of this appraisal, client and therapist then collaborate in the critic activity of assessing its adequacy. Together, they raise and consider relevant questions of various sorts. Is the self-indictment justified on empirical grounds? Is it justified on logical grounds, or is it the product of logically fallacious thinking such as overgeneralization or selective abstraction? Is it a charitable view as defined above, or does it cast the worst possible interpretation on the facts? Does it contain helpful diagnoses and prescriptions that might be used by the individual to change things? Is it the sort of thing a competent, caring parent (teacher, friend, etc.) who was attempting to act in the best interests of the person would say? If not any of these, what alternative critic acts and appraisals would meet these empirical, logical, charitable, and other criteria?

What occurs in this procedure is that therapist and client collaborate actively in the behavior of competent and constructive criticism. The benefits of such collaboration can be numerous. First, the client gains guided practice in the activity of constructive self-criticism. Second, the client derives considerable observational learning benefits from seeing a competent model engaging in this activity. Third, the situation often provides many opportunities for the therapist to acknowledge the soundness of the client's new and more adequate self-critical behaviors, thus providing a reinforcing function.

A final, perhaps less familiar benefit has to do with the fact that many persons do not feel eligible to be the definitive critics of themselves. They believe that their parents or spouses or friends surely are more competent and credible judges of them than they themselves are, and thus they tend to defer to others' judgments and mistrust their own. They fail in this way to be self-accreditors who maintain a reasonable control over their own self-esteem. The activity of serving as an increasingly competent fellow negotiator with a therapist who is perceived as highly capable in this matter can serve the invaluable function of leading clients to a new and very important conclusion: "I can be my own binding critic; I do not have to be at the mercy any longer of other critics to whom I have always deferred" (Schwartz, 1979).

USE OF TWO-CHAIR DIALOGUE EXERCISES

The great majority of clients seem to respond well to modes of talk in which the metaphors of "parts of themselves" or "subpersonalities" are employed (cf. Assagioli, 1971; Perls, Hefferline, & Goodman, 1951; Stone & Stone, 1993). The present analysis, with its notion of complementary behavioral roles of person-as-critic and person-as-object-of-criticism, lends itself well to exploiting such parts metaphors for therapeutic purposes. Further, it lends itself to the use of established techniques in which such parts are put into active therapeutic dialogues of various sorts.

The most famous, and in many respects prototypical of these techniques, is the "empty chair" exercise (Shoobs, 1964). In this exercise, clients are called upon to speak to some imaginary other who is seated in a vacant chair. The speaker and the imaginary receiver might, depending on the specific therapeutic situation, be the critic, the recipient of criticism, or a detached observer–commentator witnessing the interplay between critic and criticized. In an important variation on this technique, the client may be invited to inhabit the empty chair and to respond to the speaker, thereby creating an active, back and forth dialogue between the two "parts" (Greenberg & Higgins, 1980).

Case Illustration

Carla, a 23-year-old woman, had left her husband and baby one year previously. Subsequent to leaving, she had been involved in three serious automobile accidents, in each of which she was judged at fault by the police. She came to therapy after the last of these accidents, profoundly depressed and very fearful that her "accident-proneness" would result in her death.

In exploring the circumstances surrounding Carla's leaving her husband and child, it became clear that she had left an intolerable situation. During the two years of her marriage, she had lived in a crude, poorly insulated geodesic dome in a remote location in the mountains of Colorado. The home was without bathroom facilities, running water, or a furnace. Carla's husband left every day, and sometimes would be gone for days on end, stranding her there without a car. When this pattern had persisted through two winters, Carla became intensely dissatisfied. When she and her husband proved unable to resolve their differences, Carla stated her desire for a divorce. Her husband responded by saying that he would not stand in her way, but that she would be guilty of desertion and therefore would be unable to gain custody of their child. Carla remained several months longer because of this, but ultimately left when she found herself completely unable to tolerate the situation.

Despite the virtual impossibility of continuing any longer in her marital circumstances, Carla felt extremely worthless and self-hating for leaving. The primary source of these emotions was the fact that she had left her young child. Despite the strength of her feelings, however, she was far from recognizing that she, in the role of critic of herself, was the active perpetrator of all manner of highly degrading and devastating attacks on herself. Her entire consciousness consisted in a sense of quite abysmal feelings of personal worthlessness.

Subsequent to obtaining the above information, initial therapeutic efforts were devoted to helping Carla to recognize that she was on a daily basis functioning as an extremely degrading "hanging judge" to herself. She was indicting herself mercilessly for past sins, ignoring all mitigating circumstances, and possibly even condemning herself to death (in the form of the auto accidents). In what proved to be the critical session in her therapy, she was asked to engage in an empty chair exercise. In this exercise, she was to place "Carla" in the empty chair, to stand over her as a critic, and to state aloud the sorts of judgments she passed on her privately on a daily basis. Carla adapted readily to this directive, and delivered one of the most furious and hateful self-denunciations the author has ever witnessed. Subsequent to this exercise, during a debriefing period, Carla was able to recognize far better exactly what she was doing to herself as a critic to produce the worthlessness and depression she was experiencing. She could see, further, how in judging herself she ignored completely the mitigating circumstances of her impossible marital circumstances; how she was destroying herself rather than helping herself to figure out how to get her child back; and how as a critic she could make choices about how to treat herself.

Following this highly emotional session, Carla went home and slept for 24 consecutive hours. When she awoke, her depression had lifted. Subsequent work over the course of several months, much of which involved further empty chair work, was addressed primarily to altering her whole mode of appraising and treating herself. She experienced no further depression over the next six-month period. Unfortunately, however, she was not successful in her attempts to gain custody of her child.

HOMEWORK EXERCISE: SELF-CORRECTION

The following homework exercise is similar to other well-established ones in the cognitive–behavioral literature (e.g., DeRubeis & Beck, 1988; McKay & Fanning, 1992; Rehm & Rokke, 1988). Once the client has acquired some ideas about competent critic function such as those related above and has exhibited some facility in their use, he or she may be urged to employ them between sessions in the following manner. When clients detect that they are engaging in destructively self-critical activity, either by direct observation or by working backward from dysphoric feelings, they are to clarify for themselves the precise nature of the destructive criticism rendered. Once they have established this, they are to counteract it by employing procedures they have learned in the session. For example, they may utilize the sorts of evaluations and corrections discussed above under "collaborative negotiation," or they might consult themselves about how a competent, well-motivated parent or boss or teacher might handle the transgression in question. However they elect to do so, the key element is that they actively combat the destructive criticism by resorting to alternative means of self-appraisal.

For many clients, it is quite helpful to do this self-correction exercise aloud and not merely mentally. In one useful version, it may be suggested to them that when they have some privacy they are to "place themselves" in an empty chair and, standing above the chair and speaking as their own critic, attempt to shift to alternative critic behaviors. Thus, standing "above themselves," they might say aloud something like the following: "I have just been ripping you up pretty thoroughly, and I have gotten you feeling rather depressed and helpless. Right now, my goal is to cease doing the damaging things I have just been doing, and to try to criticize you in a much more constructive way. Here goes . . ." While some persons will be reluctant to do this exercise on grounds that it would be "sil-

ly" or "stupid," others find themselves able to do so and report benefiting greatly from such active attempts to combat their self-destructive tendencies. They report that, relative to doing the exercise
mentally, doing it aloud enables them to "put themselves into" the
exercise in a far more emotionally involved way and to remain far
more focused.

EXERCISE: "FIRST THE GOOD NEWS; THEN STOP!"

This relatively simple exercise can be surprisingly effective. Its
core is a directive to the client to take a brief period at the end of
each day, review the day's happenings, and single out those personal activities that were enjoyable, altruistic, constructive, productive,
or positive *in any way*. With regard to each activity so selected, the
further directive is to acknowledge explicitly its positive nature
(e.g., "That was a nice thing you did for Pat today," or "You really
had a good time taking the kids to the mall"). Thus, the essential
nature of the task is a self-reinforcing, self-affirming one. It is designed to counterbalance the exclusively negative self-critical focus
exhibited by many clients with an exercise that explicitly prescribes
a positive bias.

This directive, like any other, should be custom- tailored for
specific individuals. For example, Mary, a divorced criminal inves-
tigator in her early forties, was having a difficult time in bringing
herself to adopt more constructive forms of self-criticism. She had
long had a negative focus about herself that rendered it extremely
difficult for her to acknowledge anything positive about herself.
This negative attentional bias was buttressed by a belief that is was
morally wrong and egotistical to think well of oneself. However,
she was a competent critic of others, very supportive and affirming
at some times, yet honestly and tactfully critical at others. With this
in mind, the present directive was modified to accommodate her
weakness and her strength. This "good news" exercise was related
to her, but she was directed, not to affirm herself (which she could
not do), but to say to herself what she would say to her best friend if
that friend, not herself, had engaged in the positive activity. Mary
was able to implement the prescription so constructed. Furthermore, using her competence as a constructive critic of others, she
was able to extend this competence to appraising herself (aided by
some cognitive restructuring work regarding her moral reservations). Finally, without being directed to do so, Mary adopted this
task as a daily ritual that she intended to do permanently. At this

writing, she has shifted from being a depressed, extremely self-attacking individual to a generally satisfied, constructively self-critical one. While there was much more to Mary's therapy than this directive, its implementation clearly resulted in a sudden and rather marked improvement in her progress.

SUMMARY

In this chapter, a large number of therapeutic means for assisting clients to become more competent and constructive critics of themselves have been delineated. In general, these have fallen into two general categories. The first of these is the provision of access to images, concepts, and ideas that clients might utilize in becoming more competent critics. Here, the images of parent, boss, teacher, coach, and thermostat; the concepts of charity, forgiveness, and compassion; and the task analysis of the critic's job have all been discussed as vehicles for the conveyance of such understanding. The second major emphasis in this chapter has been on the extremely vital goal of getting clients to put these ideas into practice. In this connection, various in-session and out-of-session activities such as collaborative negotiation, two-chair dialogue techniques, in vivo self-correction, and the "good news" directive have all been proffered as means for helping clients to shift actively to wholly different and far more constructive critic behaviors.

CHAPTER 8

ADDRESSING RESISTANCES AND OTHER OBSTACLES

The therapeutic recommendations that have been made thus far in this book have been designed to minimize client resistance. Throughout, there has been the general endorsement of an approach in which the therapist assesses clients' existing purposes, values, and goals; designs interventions to be compatible with them; and avoids coming into conflict with them. Most importantly, the therapist demonstrates how alternative critic behaviors would better achieve the purposes the client has been trying to accomplish with maladaptive self-critical practices, and would do so without the negative consequences attendant upon those practices.

Despite our best efforts as therapists, however, most clients will present resistances to the adoption of alternative self-critical behaviors. When they are apprised of such alternative behaviors, these individuals will have genuine reservations, concerns, fears, and doubts about their adoption. While they have strong reason to try something new, in their minds they have stronger reason not to do so. In helping clients to define their reasons not to change and in responding to these reasons, the therapist can often overcome clients' resistances so that they are open to change.

In this chapter, six common client resistances will be described and some effective therapeutic responses to each of them will be related. Subsequently, three other obstacles to the adoption of new critic practices and some helpful measures for dealing with them will be presented. Unlike resistances, which are essentially strong misgivings about changing, these obstacles are factors in the individual's environment or personal characteristics that create impediments to change.

131

Before proceeding, a widely useful preliminary step should be noted. A recommended initial response to virtually all of the objections, concerns, reservations, and fears that clients present is to reflect them and to demonstrate an understanding of their intuitive, commonsense logic. Whenever possible, the individual's concern is heard and appreciated as a sensible, indeed quite plausible, one. Such an initial response, because it both increases the alliance with the client and demonstrates a correct grasp of his or her position, places the therapist in a stronger position from which to address the concern subsequently (Driscoll, 1984).

COMMON RESISTANCES TO THE ADOPTION OF CONSTRUCTIVE SELF-CRITICAL PRACTICES

"IT'S TOO WEAK TO BE EFFECTIVE"

When constructive self-critical approaches are related to some clients, they fear that these approaches will prove weak, insufficient responses for correcting their own mistakes, failures, and personal inadequacies. If they are to change such weaknesses, they believe, they must bring serious negative consequences to bear on themselves. They must "get really tough" with themselves. They must "read themselves the riot act." More humane approaches seem to them ineffectual "slaps on the wrist" that will not get the job done.

Subsequent to conveying an understanding of this concern to the client, various approaches are possible. One of these is to note for clients how the concern embodies precisely the logic behind their current approaches to themselves; i.e., that they must be extremely harsh and punitive with themselves to get results. The individual may be asked how well this approach has worked in the past and what its side effects have been. If the client responds that it has not worked very well, the possibility may be raised that it and its attendant logic should be abandoned and something else attempted instead. If the client seems reluctant to abandon this very punitive approach even though it has not worked to date, the therapist might suggest that perhaps the client needs to become even more harsh and punitive to see if such an approach could work if practiced more assiduously. A homework assignment along these lines might then be devised in which the client is urged to become even more draconian and to observe whether or not this is helpful.

Another useful approach to address this misgiving is to pose thought experiments for the client. One of the most compelling of these draws once again on the client's understanding of two-person systems: "Think of two people who want you to correct a mistake that you've made. The first of them is someone who in general treats you very well, is supportive of you, and appreciates your good points and your achievements. When you make a mistake, this person points it out to you clearly, relates the reasons why he or she believes it is a mistake, and advises a change. The second person is someone who in general treats you very poorly, never supports you, never notices anything positive about you, and reads you the riot act whenever you make a mistake. (Details here should be custom-tailored to the client's self-critical modus operandi.) Which of these two people will you be more inclined to cooperate with?" The link between self-criticism and change indeed seems to follow the logic of this example. Treating oneself well increases the likelihood that constructive action for change will follow upon self-criticism (Ossorio, 1976). Treating oneself in excessively harsh, punitive, and coercive ways increases the likelihood that the result will be consequences antithetical to change such as rebellion, depressive inertia, and a sense of personal ineligibility (Bergner, 1981).

"BUT IT'S THE TRUTH!"

Individuals frequently lock themselves into destructive self-critical scenarios by mistakenly regarding the whole matter as a truth issue. They see themselves, not as active critics, but as victims—as persons compelled by the evidence to recognize factually grounded truths about themselves. They do not choose how they see or treat themselves; they are forced by the facts to draw certain conclusions. This is epitomized by the client who, when more charitable behavior toward himself was suggested, responded that, "You don't seem to understand; the bedrock truth about me is that deep down I am a complete and utter asshole."

Two potentially helpful lines of thought may be posed to such clients for their consideration. The first of these is the general philosophical point that, while the facts may constrain what appraisals a person can make realistically, they do not dictate any uniquely correct specific appraisals. (A rock cannot be realistically regarded as an automobile, but it can be regarded as a weapon, a paperweight, a container of a geologic record, a Newtonian object, and much more.) Thus, for example, the facts do not dictate that persons systematically choose the least charitable interpretation possible of those facts (the fact that a woman is very concerned about her appearance does not dictate that we regard her as "vain" rather than "insecure about her attractiveness"). The facts do not dictate that individuals systematically choose the least functional or useful appraisal possible (the fact that a child is performing beneath his ability in school does not compel us to regard him as a "lazy bum" rather than as "resisting what he sees as parental coercion"). The facts do not dictate that persons select any given quality (e.g., beauty, brilliance, achievement, or popularity) and declare it an absolute requirement for personal worth.

The second line of thought that is helpful to many clients is captured in an aphorism: "It's not a truth issue; it's an issue of how you treat yourself." This aphorism draws their attention to the simple but crucial distinction between the facts and one's response to those facts. Even in those cases where there are undeniably negative truths about themselves for persons to contend with, these do not necessitate any particular treatment of themselves. The facts do not dictate, for example, that they be relentlessly harsh and cruel to themselves, or that they resort to self-degradation, or that they never forgive themselves. In short, the facts, however negative, do not dictate that they select responses that are fundamentally destructive of themselves and of their future ability to change unfortunate aspects of themselves.

"That's Okay for Others, but Not for Me"

Countless clients have double standards as critics. That is, while they believe that it is important to treat others such as their children and friends in constructive ways, they do not believe that they should treat themselves in such ways. Or, while they find some behavior or personal characteristic completely acceptable in others, in themselves they find it abhorrent. Such double standards, it goes without saying, present a therapeutic obstacle when one is trying to employ the sorts of two-person images cited previously. "Oh, yes," many clients will respond, "I would never think of regarding or treating my child in such a fashion, but in my case it's different." The practical upshot of such double standards is that potentially therapeutic resources possessed by the client are only available to them in their relations with others. These valuable resources are unavailable to them in their relations with themselves.

There are two general lines of response to such double standards that the author has found useful. The first of these involves making explicit something that is generally implicit in the dual standard. In cases where therapists have achieved a good therapeutic relationship with clients, and where it is clear that values of human equality and "not raising oneself up above others" are important to the individual, this response may be utilized. Clients may be informed tactfully that there is an element of grandiosity and even bigotry inherent in their double standards. That is, what they are declaring in effect is that "ordinary standards may suffice for ordinary people, but they are not good enough for the likes of me." (Compare: "Those standards are good enough for those outgroup members—you can't expect too much from the likes of them—but they are not good enough for us ingroup members.") If presented carefully to clients who are assured that the therapist is fundamentally on their side, such a move is an effective "well-poisoning" one (Driscoll, 1984; Ossorio, 1976). That is, clients' actions are redescribed or reframed for them in such a way that their incompatibility with existing personal values is made clear, thus providing them with reason to desist from the behavior in the future. In the language of the metaphor, it becomes a great deal more difficult to "drink from that well again."

The second therapeutic response to the presence of double standards is a much more open-ended one. It consists of determining individuals' idiosyncratic reasons for maintaining such standards and then addressing these. A case example may serve best to illustrate this response. Dale, a 32-year-old performing artist, reported that he accepted the homosexuality of his friends, but deplored it in himself. Further, he held himself to rather perfectionistic standards, but did not hold his friends to these. Upon questioning, it emerged that, while growing up, Dale had been subjected to a great deal of familial and peer rejection for his failure to be an athletic, assertive, well-built, "real man." In response to this, he had resolved that he would "show" his detractors. However, he recognized that doing so would require that he excel in every way that counted with them. By besting them on their own terms, he would force their acknowledgment of his superiority and their gross underestimation of him. To achieve his triumph, Dale would need to (1) repudiate his homosexuality (because it was unacceptable by others' standards) and (2) meet rather superhuman standards (in order to best everyone else). Dale's friends, however, would not have to be either heterosexual or perfect. Nothing about his agenda required that he hold them to his standards.

Once Dale had become aware in therapy of what he was doing, he was urged by his therapist not to give up his quest for a triumph over his old detractors without slow and careful consideration, since it had constituted a core life agenda for many years. However, he soon concluded that, because his quest was so painful, impossible, ultimately empty, and based on others' values, its fulfillment was a poor way to continue to expend his life energies. He abandoned this quest to show up his detractors, and with this the double standards regarding homosexuality and perfection that it had entailed. At this point, the more humane and reasonable perspectives on sexuality and perfection that he had long applied to his friends became available for application to himself.

"You're Asking Me to Settle for Mediocrity"

Many persons, when the difficulties entailed by their perfectionistic standards are brought to their attention, are quite unwilling to give up these standards. In their minds, doing so is tantamount to settling for mediocrity and abandoning the quest for personal excellence. When the therapist seems to be advocating an abandonment of their standards and promoting the adoption of more humanly achievable ones, the cure seems to them to be worse than the disease. In their minds, it is better to strive for perfection and suffer some painful consequences than to lower their personal standards and become the sort of mediocrity that the therapist seems to be suggesting.

With persons such as this, the recommended approach is not to go against their entrenched standards, which in the author's experience is a losing game. Rather, it is to show these individuls a way to keep their standards, but to use them in a new way that will better achieve their existing purposes. This approach is derived from the perspective of Niebuhr (1956) that was related previously in Chapter 3. These individuals may be shown how, with respect to their core values, they need not abandon their quest for excellence and even perfection. Their problem lies not in the standard itself, but in their treating it as a criterion of personal adequacy. Then, in the face of their inevitable failures, they damn themselves as utter failures and thus damage their ability to achieve excellence. As an alternative, they may be encouraged to treat the standard as the only thing it could be realistically: an ideal or guide star that will rarely if ever be attained, but that may nonetheless point a direction for their sincere striving. In the face of their inevitable failures, the response most conducive to achieving excellence will be, not self-abuse and degradation, but humble acknowledgment and renewed striving.

Furthermore, if clients are individuals who are striving for perfection in every area of life, they must be shown how seeking it everywhere is injurious to their ability to achieve it anywhere. If they truly desire excellence, therefore, they must learn to select a very few areas of life, based on their core personal values, in which to focus their pursuit of perfection (Hamachek, 1978). One therapist, when trying to put this matter into perspective with her clients, addresses the issue humorously by telling them that "Nobody's tombstone ever said that 'She never had any dust behind her couch.' "

"It's Morally Wrong"

Morality is an important matter for many individuals who are destructive critics of themselves. Indeed, as mentioned in Chapter 4, one of the reasons some persist in their self-lacerating ways is because they believe it is virtuous to do so and immorally egotistical to appraise themselves in more positive ways. These beliefs may be called into question profitably with such persons. The following moral questions have been, in the author's experience, the most beneficial ones to raise and to discuss with clients:

1. Is it any more virtuous to abuse and damage oneself psychologically than it is to do so physically with alcohol, tobacco, or other substances?
2. Since destructive self-criticism is so damaging to our ability to function, do we have a moral obligation to others such as our children and families not to destroy our ability to care for and relate to them?
3. Do not destructive self-critical practices fail a very critical moral test insofar as they diminish our ability to change our unacceptable behavior?
4. Is it morally acceptable to treat any human being the way the person is treating himself or herself?

By raising and exploring such questions, it is often possible to shift clients' existing motives to behave morally into the service of treating themselves more humanely and constructively.

Raising these moral issues is the only leverage possible in certain cases where clients are extremely self-hating. In these cases, when urged in the direction of alternative modes of self-criticism, the client poses a very fundamental question: "Why should I treat myself any better?" If the therapist offers a response to this question based on personal worth (e.g., "because you are a worthwhile human being and deserve better"), this means absolutely nothing to these clients because it is simply not how they regard themselves. If the therapist offers a response on the basis of consequences (e.g., "because it results in depression, low self-esteem, etc."), this too means little to such clients because they hate themselves, believe that they don't deserve any better, and may not even care greatly what happens to them. In such circumstances, if the client does subscribe to deeply held moral values, appealing to these values can be a very powerful answer to the client's question. Indeed, perceiving the immorality of destructive self-critical actions is sometimes the only thing that will provide the individual with the requisite motivation to change them.

"I'M AFRAID I'LL GET A BIG HEAD"

This is one of the more common reservations that clients have about refraining from their accustomed self-critical practices and adopting new, more constructive ones. They fear that they will become unacceptably "arrogant," "conceited," and "egotistical," and think that they are better than other people. In addition to the moral concerns already discussed, there is a consequence of such arrogance that these persons greatly fear. This is that other people will detect their high opinion of themselves, will brand them "stuck up" egotists, and will "shoot them down" and personally reject them (Driscoll, 1981, 1989). All of these constitute unbearably humiliating prospects for these self-critical persons.

Several avenues of response are often helpful here. The first of these is a clarification of what is being advocated in the present approach. Some who fear that they will become arrogant mishear what is being said and believe that the therapist is promoting a completely non–self-critical, "everything about me is wonderful," approach. Such a misinterpretation should be corrected by the therapist, and the client reminded that what is being advocated is a constructive self-critical approach in which a part of the person's job is to identify faults and mistakes and to correct these.

A second basis for clients' fears of egotism lies in the fact that one of the jobs of the critic consists in recognizing, acknowledging, and affirming one's own successes, competencies, and other positive attributes. Individuals are frightened that this will prove a route to arrogance. Several lines of response are often helpful in dispelling such fears. First of all, clients might be presented with a description of someone who is making an objective self-assessment along the following general lines: "Well, I believe that my strengths lie in X, Y, and Z and my weaknesses in A, B, and C; D, E, and F are areas of life where I don't really shine but I do okay." Such an example is helpful to pose to clients because in it we see a person who is certainly acknowledging positives, but who does not strike most observers as egotistical.

The notion of "self-efficacy beliefs" as developed by Bandura (1982, 1992) is a second, very helpful one to share with clients in the present context. These are beliefs that individuals have that they are competent at certain specific kinds of endeavors and are likely to be successful at them if they exert the necessary efforts. Clients may be informed, using scientific research as a buttress, that such beliefs are virtually indispensable if persons are to feel the personal confidence they need to undertake important things in life and to persist in them in the face of obstacles (Bandura, 1992; Cervone, 1989; Schwarzer, 1992). Thus, the critic's recognition and appreciation of positives, far from being an unacceptable egotism, is meeting very basic human needs for a sense of competency (cf. Erikson, 1963, on the vital importance of developing a sense of "industry").

A third response to clients who are concerned about making positive self-appraisals is to ask them to consider the opposite state of affairs where all positive criticism is withheld. For example, in two-person systems, where one person such as a parent, a teacher, or a boss never acknowleges or praises the good work or admirable characteristics of another, the usual results are feelings of demoralization, demotivation, futility, and failure in the latter. Thus, the argument goes, it is actually damaging to persons, including ourselves, to withhold such reinforcing consequences as praise, acknowledgment, and affirmation.

Finally, clients who are concerned about behaving in arrogant or conceited ways may be informed that it is usually destructive, persistently negative self-criticism that results in this outcome. They may be told that the sorts of narcissistic, grandiose self-displays that result in persons being branded conceited or egotistical usually result from a low self-esteem that has its roots in destructive self-criticism. Such displays are, more often than not, attempts to win the applause of others to meet esteem needs that persons are not able to supply for themselves (Kernberg, 1978). This being the case, more competent and constructive self-critical practices are, if anything, safeguards that *reduce* the likelihood of such self-aggrandizing behavior.

COMMON OBSTACLES TO THE ADOPTION OF CONSTRUCTIVE SELF-CRITICAL PRACTICES

In the sections to follow, a different kind of impediment to the adoption of constructive self-critical behaviors will be presented. Previously, discussion has centered aroung resistances—various misgivings, reservations, and fears—that clients have about new critic behaviors. Here, the impediments at issue are not so much reasons against changing one's behavior, but factors in the individual's environment or personal characteristics that create obstacles to change.

DESTRUCTIVELY CRITICAL OTHERS

As noted previously in this book, many persons with self-critical problems report that they are devastated by the criticisms of others, and find themselves helplessly defined by those criticisms. One young client, quoted in an earlier chapter, expressed this dilemma very aptly when she stated that, "When my father criticizes me, I am absolutely crushed; it's like God is speaking, and I just can't bring myself to believe anything other than what he is telling me." An important obstacle to these individuals regarding and treating themselves in more beneficial ways, then, is the fact that others in their lives are criticizing them destructively, and they find themselves unable to criticize themselves constructively in the face of this.

With such individuals, the following slogan may be employed to convey to them a useful conception of their difficulty: "Your main problem with other critics is that you always agree with them." The substance of this slogan, which should be carefully elucidated, is that clients' primary problems lie in their concurrence with the destructive criticisms of others (McKay & Fanning, 1992). It is only when they listen to others and conclude, often reflexively, that their criticisms must be correct in their substance and in their implications that they are vulnerable to being devastated and controlled by them. Barring this, they may find such criticisms bothersome or obnoxious but not binding and devastating.

An important implication of this conception is that clients have ultimate control over whether or not they will be devastated. They must provide something essential, their personal concurrence with the external criticism, or the latter is rendered relatively powerless. They are not mere pawns at the mercy of the slings and arrows of others' evaluations. Thus, if clients can find ways to cease their reflexive concurrence with the criticisms of others, these criticisms will be muted considerably in their power to devastate and control.

A helpful prescription in such cases is to recommend to clients, at a point when they have made some progress in becoming more constructive critics of themselves, that they "insert their own critic between themselves and others." If others offer a criticism, they are to employ the following general procedure in the handling of such criticism. First, they are, as a matter of the strictest policy, to suspend judgment regarding its merits. That is, they are to make every effort to catch themselves and to refrain from their customary, automatic "they must be right" response. Furthermore, they are to take the rigid stance that "That person may be right, partially right, or wrong; I will believe nothing until I have personally considered the matter; I will be the final judge." Second, they are to give the criticism the consideration due it and come to an independent, personal decision regarding its worth. Do they believe, based on their own best reflection, that the criticism has some merit or no merit at all? Third, if they make the personal judgment that the criticism has merit, they are to handle the matter of what does or does not need to be done in their own way. For the external critic, the matter may be a "federal offense" that warrants severe degradations and punishments, but this should in no way bind the individual from handling it in the new, more constructive and humane ways that he or she has been acquiring.

The central function of this prescription is the absolutely essential one of enabling persons to be their own ultimate critics. When they are successful, they retain an openness to the opinions of others, but are no longer at their mercy. Although the prescription may be described fairly simply and straightforwardly, its implementation is for most clients quite difficult. Further, it usually requires a great deal of supportive discussion about such matters as the supposed superiority or infallibility of external critics and the eligibility of the person to criticize himself or herself competently and authoritatively.

POSITIVE SELF-CHARACTERIZATIONS ARE UNTHINKABLE

In Chapter 2, it was pointed out that self-assigned degrading labels tend to become locked in and to become impervious to potentially disconfirming empirical evidence. One just is "stupid" or "unlovable" or "incapable of loving," etc., and all evidence to the contrary is dismissed, overlooked, or even assimilated to the degrading label (cf. Beck & Weishaar, 1989). The label is simply the unquestioned "given" (Roberts, 1985) about who or what one is.

Where these old, degrading self-characterizations constitute immutable and unquestioned givens, new and more affirming ones become the "unthinkable" (Roberts, 1985). Left to their own interpretive devices, individuals would simply never think to appraise themselves in more positive, accrediting ways (e.g., as intelligent, lovable, or giving). Further, when such status-enhancing attributions are made by other persons ("But Terry, you are very giving!"), the individual's response tends to be one of disbelief and incredulity: "That just couldn't be; that's just out of the question."

For example, Eleanor, a single computer programmer in her early thirties, was convinced that she was an ugly, selfish, deeply spiteful person, and that all of these characteristics rendered her profoundly unattractive to men (except as a sexual object). In the course of discussing other problems during therapy, she repeatedly made mention of a coworker, Peter, who would often stop by her desk, ask her to lunch, initiate relatively personal conversations, and in other ways behave in a manner suggesting that he found her attractive. When, however, it was suggested to Eleanor that there seemed to be considerable evidence that Peter was attracted to her, she seemed quite shocked and responded that, "No, that's completely impossible; he's just a nice guy."

Obviously, if positive self-characterizations have the status of unthinkables in a person's world, this is a significant obstacle to positive, constructive self-criticism. In such circumstances, the author has found it helpful to pursue a twofold strategy. The first element in this strategy is to make the client aware of what he or she is doing in terms of givens and unthinkables. For example, with Eleanor, the therapist approached her along the following lines. "It looks like you have a very fixed label for yourself: 'unattractive to men.' And when anything happens that would seem to contradict that label, such as Peter asking you out to lunch repeatedly, discussing personal matters with you, and hanging around your desk all the time, you conclude that this couldn't possibly mean what it looks like to everybody else—that he's attracted to you. To everyone else, such as your coworkers and now me, it looks like he is interested in you. To you right now, however, this is unthinkable; this just couldn't be. And so you look for some explanation of the evidence that is consistent with your conviction that you're unattractive: he's 'just a nice guy.' "

The essence of this move is that clients are made aware of what they are doing when they regard their old labels as the unquestioned givens, interpret apparently inconsistent evidence to fit these labels, and effectively write off as unthinkable far more plausible interpretations of events. Such a procedure will often serve to make it harder for the client to continue to interpret events in the future (e.g., Peter's next luncheon invitation) in such reflexively negative ways. Finally, the move introduces new and more status-enhancing possibilities to the client (here, "attractive to Peter").

The second part of this strategy is to assess any obstacles to the client's acceptance of new and more positive self-appraisals and to address these if found. If the client were to see himself or herself as intelligent, or lovable, or giving, would this present any problems? Would it be frightening? Would it seem unacceptably egotistical? Would it present problems in terms of the enhanced expectations of others? Would it create any other sorts of difficulties?

Perhaps the most common obstacle that is found here is that the new, more self-affirming characterizations seem to clients to be impossibilities for them. Given who they see themselves as being, these new possibilities seem quite unimaginable and impossible. It is as if one was a poor singer and was being asked to imagine himself being invited to join one of the world's great opera companies; or one was an average athlete and was being asked to imagine herself winning an Olympic gold medal. The reaction is: "Who, me? I simply cannot see myself there. I cannot imagine this as a real possibility. This is unthinkable for me."

In Eleanor's case, the following metaphor was employed to address this impasse. It embodies musical content because she had musical interests, but can be employed profitably with many clients by adapting its content to their specific interests. "Think of somebody who is a pianist and is invited to play at Carnegie Hall for the first time. She's never played at such a prestigious place, a place so renowned for its association with great musical performers. Her natural reaction on first receiving the invitation is one of disbelief: 'No, this isn't possible; this can't be me who's been invited to play at Carnegie Hall; there must be some mistake.' She has a second

natural reaction—fear. It's frightening to her, as it would be to anyone, to think of herself as about to perform on such a lofty stage.
The upshot of this 'it-couldn't-be-me' feeling and this fear is that it
takes a little time for the truth to set in that it's true, she has been invited to play there and no mistake has been made. And [to Eleanor],
I think this is where you are now. You look at this new and very
positive situation and your first reaction is to think, 'No, this is really quite impossible; I can't see myself being pursued by a man, and
especially by one who is so nice and so attractive. His attentions
can't possibly mean what they seem to mean.' And it's frightening
to think that he wants a relationship with you. Just as the pianist
wonders if she can live up to what has come her way, so do you. I
suspect that what you'll find is that the truth will settle in slowly—
you'll sort of 'grow into it'—that Peter, and other men that you may
not even be aware of now, do find you attractive."

The therapeutic endeavor here is to create a construction of reality wherein the unthinkable can become thinkable. The dynamics
of resistance to rethinking one's status in the world are explicated in
familiar, metaphorical terms. Furthermore, they are framed as understandable, universal dynamics that have nothing to do with
mental illness. Finally, it is suggested that certain facts about one's
place in the world (here, about one's attractiveness) are simply the
case and may be allowed to come in at a pace that one's fear and
one's disbelief allows. In Eleanor's case, a belief in her attractiveness and desirability to men was not established in time for her to
capitalize on Peter's interest. However, she did come to believe,
through this strategy and further cognitive work, that she was indeed attractive to him. She subsequently met another man, formed
a very good relationship with him, and married for the first time at
the age of thirty-four.

Destructively Criticizing Oneself for Being a Destructive Critic

When pathologically self-critical persons become aware of
their self-critical ways, it is only to be expected that they will often
respond to them as they have to their other faults and mistakes in
the past. They will become critical of them in destructive ways.
They will "hang the hanging judge," become perfectionistic about
being a nonperfectionist, and degrade themselves for being so de-

grading (Bergner, 1981; McKay & Fanning, 1992; Ossorio, 1976; Rubin, 1975). Such negative reactions are not entirely a bad beginning here. It is at least a strong reaction *against* what one has been doing, and is therefore preferable to other common reactions (e.g., a resigned despairing one or a resistant one). However, in the long run, this reaction is unconstructive for the obvious reason that it represents a perpetuation of the precise problem. The individual finds himself or herself in the kind of dilemma described by Alan Watts (1940) when he remarks that "the hate of hatred is only adding one hatred to another, and its results are as contrary as those of the war that was fought to end all wars" (p. 59).

Two therapeutic approaches to this obstacle have been found helpful by the author. The first of these is simply to make the client aware that he or she is employing destructive practices as a reaction against destructive practices, and thus is perpetuating rather than resolving the precise problem. Aphorisms such as "don't hang the hanging judge" (Ossorio, 1976, p. 132) can be especially useful here because they tend to stick in people's awareness and they enable the therapist to recapture the whole idea repeatedly simply by restating the aphorism. Because the reaction against pathological forms of self-criticism in such cases has been a strong one, the awareness by these clients that they are perpetuating the problem gives them significant reason to try to catch themselves in the future and desist from what they are doing.

The second response to this obstacle is to assist individuals in gaining a more charitable perspective on themselves as critics (Bergner, 1981; Stone & Stone, 1993). Their initial response has been to reject themselves as stupid, malevolent, crazy, or otherwise defective for treating themselves as they have. However, drawing on what was said in Chapter 4 about the purposes of self-criticism, clients may be helped toward a more charitable attitude. Depending on the particular case, they might be shown how as critics their intent was to secure such worthwhile goals as protecting themselves from various dangers, improving themselves, or attempting to achieve excellence. The critic is framed as analogous to a well-meaning parent who desires worthwhile things for his or her child, but has been only partially successful in finding the best ways to secure these. Such a framing provides the underpinning for a far more understanding and charitable reaction and is a powerful antidote to the initial tendency of the client to try in one way or another to "kill the critic."

CONCLUSION

In the author's experience, it is the rule rather than the exception that clients will have significant concerns, misgivings, and obstacles where changing to new critic behaviors is concerned. It is therefore incumbent upon the therapist both to be aware of these impediments and to possess some therapeutic options to address them effectively. In this chapter, therefore, a large number of such impediments, as well as therapeutic recommendations for responding effectively to them, have been described.

CHAPTER 9

THE THERAPEUTIC RELATIONSHIP IN THE TREATMENT OF PATHOLOGICAL SELF-CRITICISM

What sort of therapeutic relationship would best facilitate clients adopting more humane and constructive modes of self-criticism? The focus of this chapter will be on providing an answer to this question. Before turning directly to this answer, a general reminder of an important relationship between self-appraisal and the appraisal of other persons should be helpful to an understanding of the form that this answer will take.

PRELIMINARY CONSIDERATIONS

People will tend to appraise themselves as they have been appraised by others. This core idea has appeared over many decades in numerous highly respected psychological and sociological theories and has been supported by some empirical inquiry. To cite but a few examples, psychoanalysts (e.g., Arlow, 1989; Brenner, 1975; Freud, 1923) have long contended that the voice of the praising and prohibiting parent becomes incorporated by each person as the model for his or her self-appraisals (superego). Classical sociologists such as Cooley (1902) and Mead (1934) asserted that the feelings and attitudes of each person toward himself or herself derive primarily from the feelings and attitudes of other persons toward him or her. More recent sociological work in the area of labeling theory (Stephan & Stephan, 1990) picks up this earlier theme in its demonstrations that labels that persons attribute to themselves (especially deviant ones) tend to mirror the community's evaluations of these persons. Rogers (1951; Raskin & Rogers, 1989) contended that the type of positive regard held by parents toward their children (and later by therapists toward their clients) will be reflected in the kind of positive regard these children (and clients) will come to have for themselves. Finally, a number of empirical studies attest to the validity of the proposition that persons will come to appraise themselves as they have been appraised by others in their families of origin (e.g., Frost et al., 1991; Koestner et al., 1991).

The upshot of this relationship between the appraisals of others and self-appraisal for our present concerns is clear. The primary goal of therapy with pathologically self-critical persons is to enable them to criticize themselves more humanely, constructively, and effectively. What all of these positions and findings imply is the following: A relationship in which the therapist represents the appraising other, and in which he or she appraises the client in constructive and accrediting ways, can be a very powerful vehicle for helping pathologically self-critical clients to appraise themselves more beneficially (cf. Rogers, 1951, 1959).

ILLUSTRATION OF FORM OF THERAPEUTIC RELATIONSHIP

The present formulation of the therapeutic relationship possesses some continuity with previous characterizations of this relationship (e.g., Brady, 1980; Rogers, 1951, 1959; Wilson, 1989). When taken as a whole, however, it is markedly different from any of them. Because of this, it is perhaps best to orient the reader to the present conception with an illustration.

The 1938 film classic, *Boys' Town*, provides an excellent vehicle for conveying the form, though not the content, of the present conception of the therapeutic relationship. In this loosely biographical film, a priest, Father Flanagan, runs a community charged with the care of boys who have been in trouble with the law. His core philosophy is expressed in the motto, "There's no such thing as a bad boy." In the eyes of Father Flanagan, each new boy who enters Boys' Town is viewed, a priori, as a good boy. Furthermore, there is almost nothing the boy can do to change the priest's view of him. Should the boy misbehave in some manner, this behavior is always seen by Father Flanagan, in one way or another, as a misguided act or a bad act by a good boy. It is never taken as empirical grounds to reconsider the young man's basic goodness.

The priest's philosophy infuses all of his actions toward his boys. Not only does he view them as good, but he unfailingly treats them as such. Because the boys regard Father Flanagan as a very estimable and credible person, the priest's persistent treatment of them as good eventually leads them to view themselves as he views them. In their own eyes, they become basically good persons. Finally, with this recasting of themselves as acceptable individuals, they rethink their basic eligibilities in society. From outcast positions, they see themselves as having moved to positions of membership in society, and with this as having acquired the enhanced eligibilities for relationsips, jobs, and ways of life that go with this new position.

What is observed in this illustration is an informal version of an "accreditation ceremony" (Garfinkel, 1957; Ossorio, 1976, 1978). In this ceremony (which is the diametric opposite of the "degradation ceremony" described in Chapter 2), one person, who occupies a position of high status and credibility, regards other individuals in a highly affirming and accrediting way and treats them accordingly. This accrediting treatment proves successful in this case when the latter individuals accept the statuses assigned and come to greatly enhanced conceptions of themselves and their eligibilities to participate in society.

The positive therapeutic relationship may profitably be regarded as an ongoing, informal version of an accreditation ceremony. Its essential ingredients are as follows:

1. The therapist makes a priori status assignments to the client that are accrediting in nature.
2. The therapist treats the client accordingly.
3. The client regards the therapist as a credible status assigner.
4. The client recognizes the status assignments that are being made to him or her.
5. The client accepts the therapist's status assignments; i.e., appraises himself or herself in these ways.

In the remainder of this chapter, each of these five elements of accreditation ceremonies will be discussed in greater detail. In doing so, the considerable power and benefit of engaging pathologically self-critical clients in accrediting therapeutic relationships will be explicated.

ELEMENT 1: THERAPIST MAKES A PRIORI STATUS ASSIGNMENTS THAT ARE ACCREDITING IN NATURE

STATUS AND STATUS ASSIGNMENT

As noted in Chapter 2 in connection with degradation ceremonies, the term *status* refers to an individual's "place" or "position." The totality of a person's statuses is simply the totality of that person's positions in relation to everything. "Everything" here includes other persons, communities to which the individual belongs, elements of the inanimate world, and even himself or herself (Ossorio, 1976, 1982; Schwartz, 1979). For example, Joe may be a father to his child, a husband to his wife, a lieutenant in the armed services, a member of the Catholic religion, his own harshest critic, a strong valuer of family loyalty, and an author of his own actions, among countless other relations to himself and his world.

Each of a person's various statuses corresponds to some behavior potential (Ossorio, 1976, 1990); that is, to be in any relational position is to have greater or lesser eligibility and/or opportunity to engage in certain behaviors. For example, to hold officer's rank in the military is to be eligible to give orders to those of lesser rank, to partake in officers' club functions, and more. To be a marital partner to another ordinarily carries eligibilities and opportunities to relate sexually, to co-govern a family, to share experiences, to build a life together, and much more.

Sociological statuses such as "lieutenant" and "spouse" are especially clear instances of statuses that carry with them behavior potential. Less clear is the fact that personal attribute labels, a class of concepts usually taken as designating qualities inhering "in" persons, also designate such statuses. Charlie Brown, in the Charles Schulz cartoon cited at the outset of Chapter 2, appreciates this fact very well when he laments, "I'm a nothing, and she's a something, so I can't go over and have lunch with that pretty red-haired girl" (Schulz, 1968). Charlie Brown appreciates that his self-assigned "nothing" is not merely the description of some quality or lack thereof in himself, but also a status. This self-designation places or locates him somewhere in relation to others. In this instance, it is a place of tremendous disqualification and ineligibility for relations with them (cf. Goffman, 1963, on stigmatizing labels).

In like manner, other personal attribute concepts that persons employ to characterize themselves and others (e.g., "irrational," "honest," "trustworthy") are, when we examine them from this status perspective, seen to be not merely qualities but statuses. When we appraise Joe as an honest person, we are not merely taking it that he has a certain quality. We are also assigning him to a place or position in our worlds such that we are prepared to treat him quite differently than Jack, whom we take to be dishonest. When we appraise ourselves as "crazy" or "irrational," we assign ourselves to places that are quite different than "sane" or "rational" and we treat ourselves and our actions quite differently. For example, if we regarded ourselves as rational, we would trust our judgments far more and act on them with greater confidence than if we believed ourselves crazy.

A Priori Status Assignments

Ordinarily, we assign statuses to others on empirical grounds. We observe Joe, and on the basis of our observations, we recognize that he has the statuses "lieutenant," "father," "valuer of family loyalty," "honest," "his own harshest critic," and so forth.

However, it is possible to make status assignments a priori. A commonplace example of this occurs every day in jury trials. Jurors are instructed explicitly, prior to any observation, to regard defendants as "innocent until proven guilty." They are instructed to hold the defendant, a priori, innocent of charges until and unless the evidence presented is such that they can have no reasonable doubt but that he or she is guilty.

A second example of an a priori status assignment is more directly relevant to our present concern with positive therapeutic relationships. Rogerian and other psychotherapists, upon first meeting new clients, will assign the status "unconditionally acceptable" to them, and will treat them accordingly from the first moment that they enter the consultation room. Their position will not be the openly empirical, "Well, let's wait and see if this person seems acceptable to me." It will be the a priori, "As a human being, this person is unconditionally acceptable; I will hold him or her such to the degree that my own personal ability permits; in the face of failure to do so, my first line of endeavor will be to expand my own personal tolerance."

Accrediting Status Assignments

A status assignment is accrediting when its acceptance entails, or is equivalent to, the acceptance of expanded eligibilities and/or opportunities to participate in a community. Should Lucy, in one of her five-cent psychiatric sessions characterize Charlie Brown as a "something," and should he be able to accept this characterization as real, his acceptance would entail an appraisal of himself as eligible for relationships with others he deems worthwhile "some-things." Should a therapy client, through experiencing a relationship in which she was unconditionally accepted, come to regard herself as unconditionally acceptable, her new self-regard would carry with it a perception of herself as eligible for acceptance from others.

A status assignment is degrading when its acceptance entails, or is equivalent to, the acceptance of diminished eligibilities and/or opportunities for participation in a community. This point was discussed at length in Chapter 2.

ELEMENT 2: THERAPIST TREATS THE CLIENT ACCORDINGLY

A woman is falsely reassured that she is not going to die, but is treated as a dying person. A child is told that he is coordinated, but is treated as clumsy. A client is told that she is rational, but is treated as one who is always misreading reality. In cases such as these, there is strong reason to believe that "actions speak louder than words" (Goffman, 1959; Heider, 1958; Reeder & Fulks, 1980). Here, this would mean that the status assignment implicit in the treatment of the person "speaks louder" than verbal reassurances. It is this status assignment that is taken by its recipient as the assigner's genuine one. In cases where verbalized status assignments and those implicit in treatment of another are congruent, it is ordinarily the latter that serves as the guarantor of the authenticity of the former, and not the other way around.

Where the therapeutic relationship is concerned, it is therefore imperative that therapists not only make a priori status assignments that are accrediting in nature, but that they treat clients in a manner that is utterly consistent with these status assignments. When conditions are optimal, this process tends to occur smoothly, naturally, and automatically. We simply see our clients as acceptable, as making sense, as "somethings," etc., and naturally treat them accordingly.

When conditions are less than optimal, however, the enactment of a therapeutic relationship in which the therapist treats the client in accrediting ways may require considerable ingenuity and work. For example, a client might report that he has been sent by the courts for sexually abusing his child and, despite his facade of earnestness, it is easy to see that his attitude is quite cavalier and that he has come to therapy primarily to avoid court sanctions. The therapist's first reaction to him is nonaccepting, and this attitude will ordinarily be expressed in the therapist's behavior even if he or she tries to fake an accepting attitude. The therapist in such a case, if he or she is to be an accrediting relater, must do something to enable himself or herself to be able genuinely to regard and treat the client in an accrediting manner. He or she might, for example, actively search for a perspective on this client that would facilitate acceptance of him. This might be accomplished by asking extensively about the man's personal history, current circumstances, phenomenology, and reasons for involving his child sexually.

The key requirement for acceptance will be that the therapist be able to get an understanding of this man that will enable him or her to accept the man (without condoning or excusing away his action). The therapist may learn, for example, that the man was himself abused, that he is radically ignorant of the implications of his actions for his child, that he does care for the child, or that he has been drastically degraded as a person in other spheres of his life. Knowledge of any or all of these facts might enable the therapist to accept him better. Of course, searches for more charitable perspectives, examinations of our own untherapeutic reactions, and other measures designed to put ourselves in a more genuinely accrediting posture vis-à-vis the client will sometimes fail and we will not be able to accept certain clients.

RECOMMENDED STATUS ASSIGNMENTS AROUND WHICH TO BUILD A POSITIVE THERAPEUTIC RELATIONSHIP

In a positive therapeutic relationship with self-critical (as well as other) clients, the therapist would ideally make a priori status assignments to them that are accrediting in nature, and treat them accordingly. Where Carl Rogers would recommend that the content of such accreditation have to do with the single status "unconditionally acceptable," the current recommendation is that an accrediting therapeutic relationship be built far more comprehensively around nine statuses.

ONE WHO IS ACCEPTABLE

To be acceptable is to be eligible for the acceptance of other persons. As discussed at length in Chapters 2 and 3, countless self-critical clients have in effect declared themselves ineligible for such acceptance. By dint of assigning themselves degraded statuses (e.g., "unloving," "bad," "emotionally unstable"), appraising themselves as miserable failures vis-à-vis their own perfectionistic standards, and more, they have come to believe themselves disqualified from such acceptance. A therapeutic relationship in which the client is assigned the status "acceptable"—i.e., one in which he or she is in fact accepted by the therapist—can therefore be highly beneficial for such persons. Further, such a relationship enhances the likelihood that our other interventions will be effective, since clients are more likely to listen to and cooperate with therapists who accept them than ones who do not (Driscoll, 1984). Although their rationales are somewhat different, the vast majority of authors on the therapeutic relationship have stressed the importance of the therapist's acceptance of the client (e.g., Beck & Weishaar, 1989; Kahn, 1991; Kohut, 1977; Raskin & Rogers, 1989; Wilson, 1989).

ONE WHO MAKES SENSE

It is incalculably self-disqualifying to see oneself as making no sense. Many self-critical persons, through their second-guessing, doubt-casting, or outright dismissive reactions to themselves and their decisions, come to believe that their perceptions, emotions, judgments, and decisions are inadequately grounded in reality and/or that they are without logical foundation. When individuals continually undermine themselves in such ways, they increasingly regard themselves as unqualified for competent judgment and action. The undermining effects of such beliefs can be staggering in some cases.

In the therapeutic relationship, it is therefore recommended that the client be held, a priori, to be ineligible to make no sense. In practice, this means that the client's every emotion, judgment, and action has a logic that is in principle reconstructable, and that his or her every perception is an understandable way of looking at things. The client is eligible to be mistaken in his or her reasons, perceptions, and judgments, but not eligible to make no sense (Ossorio, 1976; Driscoll, 1984). While this status assignment has a general applicability to all clients (Bergner & Staggs, 1987), it becomes especially crucial in those cases where we are seeking to help persons to free themselves from reflexive acceptance of the criticisms of others and to become their own binding critics. If such persons are to achieve this, it is absolutely essential that they possess a basic faith in the realism and soundness of their own perceptions, judgments, and decisions.

Before leaving this status assignment, a few brief comments seem in order regarding its application to psychotic individuals. First, the policy could not be applied in those cases where there are strong grounds for believing that the etiology of symptoms is primarily biological (see, e.g., Crow, 1989, on Type II schizophrenia). Second, aside from such cases, there is a substantial literature attesting to the social intelligibility of psychotic behavior that is quite helpful in elucidating its sense (e.g., Bateson, Jackson, Haley, & Weakland, 1956; Bergner, 1985; Haley, 1980; Laing, 1965; Selvini-Palazzoli et al., 1989; Wechsler, 1993). Where the therapist is sensitive to the meanings and strategic implications of so-called "crazy" behavior, he or she will be able to respond to such behavior in a more understanding, and thus more competent fashion. For example, one psychotic young man, on being exhorted by his therapist to "have a nice Christmas," responded to her by saying "Francis Gary Powers" (Geyer-Heinrich, personal communication, 1982). The therapist who recognizes this as a veiled positive wish (Francis Gary Powers was the American pilot implicated in the famous 1960 U-2 incident—thus "you too!") is in a better position to respond sensitively and appropriately than another therapist who might dismiss the young man's rejoinder as nonsensical "word salad."

One Whose Best Interests Come First in Relationship

Generally, persons who assign to themselves the status "unlovable" take it that they are not persons whose best interests could constitute the genuine concern and goal of another. If others' action toward them seem positive, it cannot be because those others truly care about them and their best interests, and they will tend to generate alternative explanations of such events (e.g., the other person "must want something"). In contrast, persons who believe they are lovable appraise themselves as eligible or worthy to have their best interests constitute the genuine concern and goal of other persons.

It is recommended, therefore, that the therapist assign to the client the status of "one whose best interests come first in this relationship." In practice, this means that the therapist's fundamental commitment is to conduct therapy first and foremost for the benefit of the client, not the benefit of society, the client's family, the therapist, or any other party (Driscoll, 1984; Ossorio, 1976). Such a therapeutic stance is an accreditation in which the status assignment has to do with lovability. That is, it has to do with a genuine investment on the part of another human being in the client's best interests (cf. Kahn, 1991).

ONE WHO IS SIGNIFICANT

To be insignificant is to be, like Charlie Brown, a "nothing" living in a world of "somethings" and to suffer the relational ineligibilities that he so aptly described. It is to be an unimportant "nobody," a "cipher," in a world peopled by important "somebodies" (cf. Mizer, 1964). It is to live in an "I don't count—you count" world. To assign to the client a place of genuine importance and significance in one's life, then, is an accreditation. In the author's experience, such actions as sending letters to clients (e.g., when there has been a misunderstanding or for strategic purposes), making phone calls to them (e.g., with a homework assignment thought of after a session), and mentioning to the client that one was thinking about him or her during the week, are all potent therapist actions that convey to clients that they are not just one's "three o'clock appointment."

ONE WHO IS AN AGENT

Numerous clients hold implicit views of themselves in which they are helpless pawns of internal or external forces. They convey this in expressions like "something came over me," "I found myself doing such and such," "so-and-so made me do it," and the like; and these expressions permeate their descriptions of their actions. They convey this further when they portray themselves as helpless in the face of their "impulses," of their long-standing habitual patterns, of their personal histories, or of their "natures." A "pawn of forces" (e.g., a puppet or a robot) is ineligible to engage in deliberate action. "It" is incapable of entertaining behavioral options and choosing from among them. It is powerless.

In contrast, to be an agent is to be eligible to entertain behavioral options and to choose from among them. To be an agent is to have control, albeit imperfect, of one's behavior. To be an agent is to have power. Thus, personal agency is included among the a priori status assignments that it is important to include in the therapeutic relationship with self-critical (as well as other) clients.

ONE WHO IS TO BE GIVEN THE BENEFIT OF THE DOUBT

Within bounds of realism, therapists have options as to how to construe their clients. And these options differ in the degree of charity that they embody (see Chapter 7 for a fuller discussion of this concept). For example, a mother who is overly concerned about her child's safety might be viewed by a psychotherapist either (1) as someone who harbors an unconscious hatred of her child, or (2) as someone who is utterly convinced that, for her, nothing so good as her child and their relationship can possibly be lasting. The relational recommendation here is: Treat the client as one who is to be given the benefit of the doubt (Ossorio, 1976). Given a choice among different ways of looking at a client, choose as a matter of policy the most charitable yet realistic possibility.

ONE WHO HAS STRENGTHS

An individual who possessed no strengths—no enabling abilities, traits, ideas, motives, or positions of power—would be a completely helpless individual. He or she would not be qualified for the essential business of acting to better his or her own life. He or she would be eligible for the help of other, but not for self-help. The therapist who undertook therapy with the implicit assumption that "This client is a helpless person, and I shall have to proceed from there" would be starting from an almost impossible position.

It is recommended, therefore, that the therapist take it a priori that each client possesses strengths—that he or she possesses enabling abilities, traits, ideas, motives, roles, and/or positions of leverage (Driscoll, 1984). The therapeutic task here is one of finding, recognizing, and mobilizing strengths, not determining whether or not they exist.

ONE WHO IS THE THERAPIST'S ALLY AND COLLABORATOR

Being a member of a two-person community in which both persons are pulling together and collaborating to accomplish a common goal is ordinarily accrediting in two ways. First, if the therapist is an estimable person for the client, to be related to such an estimable person as his or her ally and collaborator is itself status enhancing. Second, as the old aphorism "two heads are better than one" implies, working in collaborative alliance with another is usually more enabling than working alone. Thus, treating the client as an ally and as a collaborator is recommended (cf. Beck & Weishaar, 1989; Driscoll, 1984; Sweet, 1984).

"A priori status assignment" has a somewhat different meaning here than it does elsewhere. Where alliance is concerned, one does not assume at the outset that the client is an ally, in the same sense that he or she is acceptable or sense-making. Rather, the suggestion is that the therapist initiate the sorts of behaviors toward the client that one would initiate with an ally, thus inviting and encouraging the client to enact reciprocal role behaviors (compare: making the opening move in a board game). The client may respond by immediately enacting the complementary role, thus establishing an immediate alliance. Or the client may not do so, thus necessitating additional efforts to establish the alliance.

ONE WHO IS ELIGIBLE TO ASSIGN STATUSES TO THE THERAPIST

All that has been said thus far in this chapter could be read as suggesting that the therapist "hands down" statuses from "on high"—that he or she hands them down from a position that is superior to that of the client. This is not the spirit in which all of this is intended. In fact, to enact these status assignments in that spirit would have degrading implications.

An important way to avoid such an enactment of the therapeutic relationship is to regard the client as a fellow status assigner who is eligible to assign statuses to the therapist (cf. Roberts, 1985, on mutual status assignment in I–Thou relationships). The recommendation here is that therapists listen carefully and give due consideration to the opinions, views, and reactions of clients towards them, and not permit themselves to become overly insulated from these (cf. Kahn, 1991). Such insulation can occur, for example, where therapists misuse the notion of transference in such a way that clients' reactions to them are routinely dismissed as "transference distortions."

CONCLUSION

In suggesting that all of these status assignments be implemented, there is no implication that all pathologically self-critical persons feel degraded in all of these ways. Clearly, they do not. However, even in those cases where they do not feel so degraded, to eliminate any one of these status assignments from the therapeutic relationship would be a serious mistake. For example, even if a client already believed herself acceptable (or sense-making, significant, possessed of personal agency, etc.), we would obviously be remiss if we regarded and treated her as unacceptable (irrational, insignificant, helpless to control her own behavior, etc.). The elimination of any of the relational elements listed above presents the danger of a countertherapeutic, degrading relationship between therapist and client in which self-assigned statuses that the client possessed initially might be undermined by the therapist's degrading treatment. Such a circumstance would create a risk of serious iatrogenic harm.

ELEMENT 3: THERAPIST MUST BE ELIGIBLE TO BE A STATUS ASSIGNER

In order to function effectively as a status assigner, the therapist must be eligible in the client's eyes to do so. Father Flanagan could successfully assign the status "good boy" only by virtue of his position in the eyes of his boys. In like manner, therapists can effectively assign the statuses listed in the previous section only if they are seen by their clients to possess certain requisite statuses. The most important of these therapist statuses are the following five.

CREDIBLE

If the therapist's status assignments are to be believed, the client must find him or her believable (Brady, 1980; Driscoll, 1984; Frank, 1963; Wilson, 1989). In the present context, this means that the client must regard the therapist as an honest and competent status assigner. Therefore, lying, self-denigration, lack of professionalism, incessant positiveness (who believes a movie critic who likes everything?), undue tentativeness, and other actions that would undercut the therapist's credibility must be avoided.

His or Her "Own Person"

It is important for clients to see their therapists as their "own persons." That is, they need to see them as persons who are able and willing to state their true positions on things, to agree or disagree, to cooperate or confront, and to set self-respecting limits on what they will do and will not do in relation to the client. Where this is absent (e.g., where the therapist is perceived as having to be perpetually nice and agreeable), the therapist's reactions to the client will not be perceived as legitimate affirmations of the client's status.

One Who Is Eligible to Criticize the Culture

The therapist would ideally be, in the eyes of the client, one who is eligible to criticize and even to disqualify the culture as a legitimate assigner of certain statuses. As noted in Chapter 4, many self-critical persons have accepted societal standards that are very debilitating in nature. The society has told them in effect that they must be married, heterosexual, white, high-achieving, and much more or they may not consider themselves worthwhile. Thus, it is important that clinicians position themselves to undermine these rather inhumane, unjust, and often impossible standards.

One good path for therapists to achieve this is by themselves espousing the higher and more enduring values of the culture. A lesson may be learned here from Edward Albee, the playwright, who is an effective critic of America largely because he criticizes it in terms of its own original values. Therapists who make appeals to values such as justice, integrity, authenticity, and responsibility present themselves in doing so as subscribers to the highest values of a culture. Other things being equal, they will function thereby as more effective critics of that culture in its unreasonable status-assigning practices.

If the therapist can lay claim to such a position, he or she is empowered to do two things. First, he or she may engage in cultural criticism and disqualification. For example, with a female incest survivor, the therapist may successfully undermine the cultural status assignment that says, "You are a devalued, tainted person because you have had sexual contact with your father, even though it was against your will." Second, the therapist may act from this position to accredit the client as one who also can disqualify the culture in its unreasonable status-assigning practices. To pursue the same example, when the therapist negotiates with the incest survivor the fairness and reasonableness of regarding herself as a discredited person, the therapist treats her as someone who is herself eligible to undermine unreasonable cultural status assignments (Bergner & Staggs, 1987; Schwartz, 1979).

One Who Knows the Client

Therapist accreditations can be dismissed by clients if they believe that the therapist does not really know or understand them. It is easy and commonplace for clients to dismiss accreditations with the following logic: "If my therapist really knew me, he (she) wouldn't find me so acceptable (rational, significant, etc.)." Thus it is imperative that clients be known and know that they are known in order to be able to assign to their therapists the status of "one who really knows and understands me." This point was made long ago by Carl Rogers (1957).

One Who Embodies the Statuses
Being Assigned

To accredit clients effectively in the ways that were described above, it is important that the therapist be perceived by the client as possessing these same statuses. Thus, it is important that the therapist be seen by the client as an acceptable, rational, significant, care-meriting person if that therapist is to be able to bring about these accreditations (cf. Brady, 1980). Should the therapist be regarded by the client as unacceptable, or irrational, or insignificant, these perceptions will detract from the therapist's eligibility to enact these accreditations. For example, a therapist might be seen as deficient in rationality because he or she makes judgments, not on the basis of what seems to the client to be realistic and logical, but on the basis of a theory that appears to the client bizarre and implausible. In such a circumstance, the perceived irrationality of the therapist will detract greatly from his or her ability to function as a potent status assigner.

RECOVERING FROM CLIENT DISQUALIFICATIONS

In the preceding paragraphs, discussion has focused on establishing and maintaining certain statuses in the eyes of clients. Despite therapists' best efforts, however, clients will at times disqualify them as legitimate status assigners; i.e., will devalue them as unacceptable, unbelievable, irrational people. At such times, it is imperative that therapists recognize what has happened and take measures to try to restore their own lost status. Otherwise, both therapist and client lose.

For example, some clients will devalue and disqualify a therapist precisely because the latter accepts them. The logic of this devaluation is the same as that of W. C. Fields, who in one of his movies rejected an invitation to join a club on grounds that he would never consider joining any club that would have the likes of him for a member. With a client who disqualifies the therapist on such grounds, the therapist might attempt to recover his or her lost status by relating this W. C. Fields anecdote. This story will often give the client a necessary insight to question and to undo his or her devaluation of the therapist (Ossorio, 1976).

ELEMENT 4: CLIENT MUST RECOGNIZE THE STATUS ASSIGNMENTS BEING MADE

Clients must recognize that they are being treated as acceptable, rational, significant, and so forth if accreditation is to take place. This does not mean that clients need be fully aware and fully able to articulate the nature of these status assignments. But if they remain totally unaware of them, then there is no possibility of accepting them and no possibility of accreditation and enhanced behavior potential.

It is incumbent on the therapist, therefore, to pay some attention to whether or not such recognition is occurring. The best policy here is to assume that the client is recognizing how he or she is being treated, unless there are clear indications to the contrary. Rather than look for every little positive indication, we undertake a far more manageable task: we watch for indications that our status assignments are not registering and then take appropriate action.

For example, we might get intimations from a client whom we truly accept that our accepting actions toward him are regarded as role behavior only, as "acting like therapists are supposed to act" and little more. The client is not recognizing that in this relationship he is truly accepted. In such circumstances, the therapist must do something to change this state of affairs. For example, he or she might address the matter directly: "It seems that your view of yourself is such right now that it's hard to believe that I, or anyone, might actually accept you. You look at my behavior and you think, 'Well, he's acting accepting because that's the way therapists are supposed to act. It couldn't possibly mean that he genuinely accepts me.' Now, there is no way to prove anything here, but I'd like to suggest that you watch for something. As you feel increasingly better about yourself, I'd like you to notice whether or not it will come through more and more that I'm not just playing a role here, that my acceptance of you is just that—acceptance of you." This remark, like the W. C. Fields anecdote, represents an attempt to help the client to see what he is doing, and therefore creates the possibility of his questioning and rethinking it. Further, it doesn't force anything on the client, suggests that general therapeutic progress will occur, and poses an expectation that the fact of acceptance will "come through."

ELEMENT 5: CLIENT MUST ACCEPT ACCREDITING STATUS ASSIGNMENTS

An accreditation is not complete until the status assignment is accepted by the client. Just as a job promotion may be refused, an Academy Award turned down, or a proposal of marriage refused, a therapist's accreditation may be rejected. The accreditation is then incomplete and as yet unsuccessful.

In such circumstances, it is incumbent on therapists to try to determine why status assignments have not been accepted and to do what they can to have them accepted. Has the client simply assimilated all that has gone on to his or her degrading conceptions of self (e.g., concluded that, "It's amazing how even a reject like me can be accepted by some people")? Has the client not accepted the new statuses because they seem too threatening ("If I took it that I made sense, was really in control of my behavior, and had strengths, people would expect a lot more of me and hold me accountable—that is a frightening prospect")? Has some key evidential basis for the current devalued status assignment been left untouched ("If my therapist knew about my abortion, she wouldn't be so accepting")? Has the client recognized that acceptance of the therapist's accreditations would create troublesome dislocations in other key relationships (e.g., "If I took it that my best interests did indeed count, would this jeopardize my relationship with my rather domineering and narcissistic spouse?"). These and numerous other possibilites, many of which are suggested by considerations in the preceding chapters of this book, might be examined and, when they prove fruitful, acted on to remedy them and bring accreditation to completion.

FINAL CONSIDERATIONS

The Danger of External Disconfirmation

As a general rule, it is desirable to accredit clients in such a way that other people are either unlikely or unable to disconfirm the new status. Two considerations are suggested in this regard. First, will the status assigned to a client be supported, or at least not disconfirmed, by others in his or her world? If so, we may proceed. Second, if external disconfirmation seems likely, what procedures may be employed to help insulate the client from such disconfirmation?

An example of such an attempt to insulate the client from external criticism occurred in the case of a young woman, Jill, who had long appraised herself as unlovable. This appraisal was based primarily on a childhood in which she was scapegoated by both of her parents and grossly rejected by her very narcissistic mother. Further, continued rejection and blame at the hands of her mother were currently serving to perpetuate Jill's conviction of unlovability. Aside from simply accepting Jill and putting her best interests first in the therapeutic relationship, Jill's therapist worked very hard to devise measures to render her more immune to her mother's degradations. A picture of reality was strongly and repeatedly promoted in which Jill was portrayed as a "placeholder" in her family of origin. That is, she was someone who, regardless of her own merits or value, occupied a certain position in that family such that no matter who occupied it, that person would be scapegoated. Further, the simple notion that her rather disturbed mother could not love, and that her failure to love Jill was therefore not in any sense a comment on Jill's lovability, was promoted over and over again in various ways throughout the therapy. In time, through these efforts to insulate Jill from her mother's degradations, she became relatively immune to them. Ultimately, both through the establishment of an accrediting therapeutic relationship and through these efforts to disqualify her mother as a legitimate external critic, Jill was able to appraise herself as lovable and acceptable to others. Furthermore, she was able to act on this by entering into a new relationship with a boyfriend and a better relationship with her father.

ENACTING THE THERAPEUTIC RELATIONSHIP IS AN INTERVENTION

A classical issue in the field of psychotherapy concerns the relative importance of the therapeutic relationship as opposed to therapeutic interventions in affecting change. Four general positions have been taken on this issue. First, some theorists, most notably those with a client-centered orientation (e.g., Raskin & Rogers, 1989; Rogers, 1957, 1959), have maintained that the therapeutic relationship is by itself both necessary and sufficient to bring about therapeutic change. Second, certain behaviorists (e.g., Lang, Melamed, & Hart, 1970) and cognitive theorists (e.g., Ellis, 1984) have held essentially the opposite view—that a positive therapeutic relationship is neither necessary nor sufficient to produce therapeutic change. A third position, entertained by other cognitive (e.g., Beck et al., 1979) and behavioral theorists (e.g., Sweet, 1984) is that a positive therapeutic relationship represents a precondition—a sort of necessary, enabling, but itself noncausal medium—for therapeutic change. Fourth and finally, most psychoanalysts (e.g., Arlow, 1989; Kohut, 1977) and certain behavioral theorists (e.g., Lazarus, 1980; Liberman, 1969) have maintained that the enactment of a positive therapeutic relationship is itself a change-producing intervention, but one that in most cases must be supplemented by further interventions to produce therapeutic change.

The present position is consistent with this last one. It is that the enactment of an accrediting therapeutic relationship as described above is itself an intervention—is something a therapist does to bring about therapeutic change. The therapist's relational behavior is instrumental behavior with a therapeutic end. As such, it qualifies as an intervention every bit as much as correcting a misconception or doing systematic desensitization. It is simply a subset of the set of all interventions in which the therapist engages.

Though a subset, this is a necessary subset. The author's experience has been that, when an accrediting therapeutic relationship does not develop, positive therapeutic outcomes rarely ensue (cf. Brady, 1980). The relative absence of such a relationship results both in failures to accredit the client and also in lessened effectiveness for other attempts to enable the client to criticize himself or herself in more humane and constructive ways.

Finally, because our primary interest has been in therapeutic change, we have discussed the therapeutic relationship only insofar as it is instrumental in bringing about certain goals. In so discussing it, the intention is not to minimize the fact that such a relationship also embodies certain ethical values (e.g., the Kantian injunction to treat every person as an end and not as a means). Nor is there an intention to minimize the fact that the relationship described has intrinsic value as a personal relationship. It is, for those who can appreciate it, an end in itself and not merely a means to some further end (cf. Roberts, 1985).

MODIFYING THE RELATIONSHIP FOR SPECIFIC CLIENTS

It is not recommended that therapists alter the nature of the status assignments made for different clients. On the other hand, it is recommended that they alter the mode of expression of these status assignments (cf. Beck et al., 1979; Bergner & Staggs, 1987; Brady, 1980). For example, where one might be relatively warm and forthcoming in one's expressions of acceptance for many self-critical clients, one would be ill-advised to do so with some others. The latter might be clients, for example, who would feel vulnerable and frightened with a therapist who approached them in this way. The need in such cases is to find ways to convey acceptance that would not threaten or provoke any other untoward reaction in these individuals. The adoption of a more formal, professional stance in which acceptance would be conveyed in the therapist's descriptions of the client would represent one such way. Without multiplying examples, the general point here is that the way in which a status assignment is conveyed must take into account the personal characteristics of the client if we are to be successful accreditors.

CONCLUSION

A very powerful supplement to all of the techniques mentioned in previous chapters of this book is to enact them in the context of an accrediting therapeutic relationship. In this relationship, the therapist assigns to the client certain a priori statuses of a highly affirming, entitling nature and treats the client accordingly. These statuses include: one who is acceptable, who makes sense, whose best interests come first, who is significant, who possesses strengths, who is to be given the benefit of the doubt, who is an ally and collaborator, who is an agent, and who is eligible to assign statuses to the therapist.

In order for clients to accept these status assignments, they must regard the therapist as eligible to make them. Thus, therapists must present themselves as credible, as their own persons, as subscribers to the best and deepest of the culture's values, and as embodying the statuses they are themselves assigning. Finally, therapists must attempt to assess and to remove any barriers to clients' recognition and ultimate acceptance of accrediting status assignments.

The positive therapeutic relationship is a powerful intervention in cases of pathological self-criticism. When enacted well, it provides enormously powerful external support and confirmation for clients' efforts to appraise themselves more positively and constructively. Finally, it provides a corrective developmental experience. Degraded historically in other important relationships, the individual is accredited in this one. Harshly and punitively indicted in others, the individual is approached with charity in this one. Held to impossible standards in other relationships, the individual is found successful by human standards in this one.

CHAPTER 10

ENCOURAGING
COMMITMENT

The solemn, deep promise to be gentle with ourselves must be
invoked again and again.

T. I. RUBIN (1975, p. 27)

When individuals are able to abandon pathological self-critical
practices and to adopt more constructive ones, the consequences for
their lives are pervasive and significant. Some of these consequences, summarized from previous chapters, include the following:

- Their self-esteem—their summary appraisal of their own
  goodness, worth, and value—is enhanced.
- Their sense of eligibility for valued relationships, jobs, and
  other life opportunities is increased, and with it their sense
  of freedom and ability to act to acquire such things. They no
  longer feel restricted or paralyzed by self-critical acts that in
  the past had left them feeling disqualified from the pursuit
  of these things.
- They are less vulnerable to being devastated and controlled
  by the criticisms of other persons. Having assumed control
  of their own critical appraisals in constructive ways, they no
  longer automatically concur with the destructive ones offered by others. Not only does this render them less vulnerable to devastation, but it also leaves them less dependent
  on others for their esteem and more able to steer their own
  course in life unfettered by an inordinate concern with what
  others might think of them.

- Having ceased their exclusively negative self-critical focus, they can now recognize, acknowledge, and appreciate positive things about themselves. They are thus able to derive vital senses of personal efficacy, accomplishment, and satisfaction that come with such self-recognitions.
- They are more able to make changes in themselves when such changes are needed and possible. No longer engaged exclusively in forms of criticism that undermine their ability to change, they are more able to generate usable problem diagnoses, implementable prescriptions for change, and new behaviors consistent with these.
- They are freer from painful and debilitating emotional states that result from destructive self-criticism and its behavioral sequelae. Most frequently, these have included depression, anxiety, guilt, and shame.
- Finally, no longer so exclusively obsessed with the dire necessity to achieve certain outcomes (since the critic will no longer use unfortunate ones as ammunition to wreak havoc), they are more able to relax and enjoy the process of immersed participation in life.

ENCOURAGING COMMITMENT

With so much at stake—so many consequences affecting so many vital areas of living—it is of inestimable benefit to clients to maintain the constructive self-critical perspectives and behaviors that they have acquired in therapy. However, in the author's experience, some clients will achieve many of these gains, maintain them for weeks and even months, and then return to their old modes of self-criticism. While some means for preventing such regressions have already been related in Chapter 5, one additional means will be discussed here in concluding this book. This is the therapeutic procedure of encouraging clients to make a deep personal commitment to continue the new self-critical perspectives and practices that they have acquired.

Posing the Idea of a Personal Commitment

Rubin (1975), in his psychoanalytic treatise, Compassion and Self-Hate, advocates that compassion toward oneself be made a personal "way of life" (p. 145). Such compassion, he contends, is central to the achievement of a life marked by joy, meaningful participation, and freedom from the many dire consequences of self-hate. Thus, he argues, it behooves individuals to commit themselves to the adoption of a personal philosophy whose centerpiece is a compassionate approach to oneself. For Rubin, the utilization of such an approach should not be left a one-time, temporary, or piecemeal matter. It should, like other core life commitments, constitute an abiding "solemn, deep promise" (p. 27) to treat oneself in such a way.

Echoing Rubin, it is beneficial to conclude successful treatment of pathological self-criticism with explicit encouragement of the client to make a deep and lasting personal commitment. This commitment is to continue to treat himself or herself in the more humane and constructive ways that have been acquired through therapy. If the client has been able to achieve positive change through the adoption of a concept (e.g., "charity" or "compassion") and/or an image (e.g., "parent" or "boss"), the link between such adoption and such change should be made painstakingly clear. If he or she has benefited from behavioral procedures (e.g., "self-correction" or "first the good news"), again the connection between this behavior and improvement should be clarified. Subsequent to such clarifications, it should be stated explicitly that continued employment of these ideas and practices is essential to continued success. Therefore, the making of a deep personal commitment to such continuance will be of great benefit in maintaining therapeutic improvements.

In a manner similar to Beck and his associates (Beck et al., 1979; Beck & Emery, 1985; Beck & Weishaar, 1989), the basic message here to the client is the following: "You have learned something of immeasurable benefit in helping yourself, and it is in your best and lasting interest to commit yourself to its continued use in your life. The kinds of events (mistakes, failures, imperfect performances, etc.) that have caused you in the past to degrade and crucify yourself will recur. If you can dedicate yourself to responding to them in the future with the perspectives and behaviors that have served you well during the course of therapy, you will have made an enduring, basic change in your life."

USING COMMITMENT SLOGANS AND STATEMENTS

Various organizations help their members to maintain vital personal commitments through the use of slogans and statements.

The function of such devices is generally to remind members of beneficial ideas and commitments and to help them to renew their dedication to them. For example, in Alcoholics Anonymous, members often employ the slogan, "One day at a time," to remind themselves of a perspective on their personal efforts that frames them in a far more manageable, less overwhelming way. In the same organization, longer and more complex reminders such as the "serenity prayer" and the "twelve steps to recovery" may be recited periodically in order to renew a personal resolve to pursue the path of sobriety. In much the same way, such slogans and statements of personal dedication may be employed by persons in their efforts to eschew pathological forms of self-criticism and to embrace constructive ones.

Slogans

Various slogans, mottos, aphorisms, and maxims may be recommended to clients or may be devised by them personally. In keeping with the general therapeutic policies advocated throughout this book, such slogans should be tailored to specific clients. Ideally, the slogan prescribed would be a crystallization of the primary solution that has worked for this client and would capture the ideology or perspective behind this solution. Other considerations may include tailoring the specific language, degree of sentimentality, and favored images or metaphors to the specific client. Designing or selecting such slogans carefully will enhance the likelihood that they will intrigue and captivate clients and will be adopted by them as a very economical means for recapturing a complex solution and for renewing their personal commitment to it.

Some slogans or mottos that have been employed beneficially by the author in his clinical work include the following:

- "Criticism is for the benefit of the actor."
- "Never destroy."
- "Perfection is a guide star, not a destination."
- "I categorically refuse to embark on flights of self-hate for any reason whatsover" (from Rubin, 1975, p. 150).
- "Your problem with other critics is that *you* agree with them."
- "My job (as a critic) is to take care of you."
- "My job (as a critic) is to be a good parent to you."

Commitment Statements

A commitment statement is similar to a slogan in that it is a highly condensed vehicle for crystallizing an important perspective or solution into few words. Further, like a slogan, it is designed to be recited by the individual as a reminder and as a reaffirmation of commitment. Such a statement may be memorized or it may be written on a small card and kept in the client's wallet or purse for easy access. It may be recited each morning, each evening, or on any other schedule found to be helpful. It should never be read passively, but always in a spirit of reaffirmation and rededication to its content.

Such a commitment statement was written for Daniel, the architect who has been mentioned several times previously in this book. The final version was the result of a first draft by the author and subsequent revisions by Daniel. Some of the original considerations that went into designing the statement were that Daniel (1) was very ethically oriented; (2) was a competent and dedicated father of three children; (3) had problems primarily with the self-degradation and "hanging judge" varieties of self-criticism; and finally, (4) had an affinity for a William Butler Yeats poem entitled *A Deepsworn Vow* (in Drew & Connor, 1961, p. 211). The commitment statement, essentially a promise to himself to be a certain kind of self-critic, read as follows:

> Today, my job—indeed my moral commitment and deepsworn vow—is to take care of you, as a good parent takes care of his child. It is to notice, acknowledge, and appreciate your strengths, accomplishments, enjoyments, and moral actions. It is also to notice and to acknowledge when things have gone wrong. When these are correctable, I will try to correct you without degrading you or attacking you viciously, remembering that this only destroys you and does not help you to change anything. When they are not correctable, I categorically refuse to take your personal limitations and failings and use these as ammunition to destroy you.

Daniel kept a written copy of this commitment statement on a small card in his wallet. He began each day by reading it and thereby renewing his "deepsworn vow" to himself. He combined this with the daily practice of the "first the good news" exercise (Chapter 7) at bedtime and with the occasional employment of the "self-correction" exercise (Chapter 7) if he found himself becoming depressed or unusually upset. The combination of these practices resulted in Daniel remaining free of his previous depressions over what is now a two-year period.

A SUMMING UP

At this point, our delineation of a comprehensive approach to the assessment and treatment of pathological self-criticism has been completed. In order to assist the reader in pulling together what has been stated over the course of many chapters, the primary procedures entailed in this approach will be summarized in closing.

ASSESSMENTS

Assess Pathological Practices

Assess the precise nature of the destructive self-critical practices that the client is employing. Do so in such a way that, not only does the clinician learn their nature, but the client becomes acutely aware of what he or she is doing. In addition to standard interviewing techniques, having the client self-monitor, interviewing him or her in the role of self-critic, and logically reconstructing the nature of self-critical acts from their effects all represent effective ways to obtain this information.

Assess Ownership of Self-Critical Behaviors

Assess the degree to which clients fully recognize that they are the perpetrators of self-critical actions. Do they recognize this or do they experience the behavior as somehow inflicted on them by sources that seem beyond their control ("My critic won't let me alone")? To change, clients must ultimately assume a position of recognized personal authorship and control over self-critical actions.

Assess the Client's Purposes

Assess what the client is attempting to accomplish with his or her pathological self-critical behavior. Is it self-improvement, atonement for past misdeeds, the achievement of safety from the dreaded reproaches of others, or other objectives? Recognize that pathological practices are usually only marginally successful at achieving their intended purposes, and that they always achieve them at grave personal costs. Thus, knowledge of these existing motivations may be used to interest the client in far more effective and less costly ways to secure their purposes, i.e., in constructive modes of self-criticism.

Assess Problematic Situations

Determine those situations in which clients seem most prone to engage in pathological self-criticism. Do they experience particular difficulties on reception of criticism from others, the mere presence of impressive others, personal failures or setbacks, stressful situations in general, and/or losses of control in personally sensitive areas? Again, not only clinicians but also clients should become aware of such troublesome situations. Being sensitized to them and to their customary self-critical reactions, clients are thereby better able to recognize these danger situations when they occur and to avoid falling into their previous automatic response patterns.

Assess Historical Influences

Assess relevant historical influences on clients' current self-critical behavior. Were degrading labels attributed to them in their families of origin, resulting in a lasting acceptance of such labels and a tendency to attribute them unquestioningly to self? Were present modalities of self-criticism such as perfectionism modeled in the family of origin, again leading to a reflexive acceptance of them as "the only way to think?" Assess especially historical factors that heuristically suggest useful therapeutic interventions in the present.

HELPING CLIENTS ABANDON PATHOLOGICAL PRACTICES

Prescribe Pathological Practices

Prescribe the continuance of the client's existing self-critical behavior. However, simultaneously prescribe an entirely different mode of perpetration of that behavior designed to give the client far more control over it and far more ability to make an ultimate choice regarding its continuance. The previous mode of perpetration of pathological self-critical behaviors has typically been instantaneous, automatic, and nonreflective. By prescription, the behavior is now to be engaged in consciously and deliberately. Further, it is to be accompanied by an investigative, observational stance wherein the client focuses on such matters as (1) whether the behavior is achieving its intended purposes, (2) what advantages and disadvantages it carries with it, and (3) what fears are raised when its discontinuance is contemplated. Finally, it is to be engaged in under a new prohibition against changing it. The client is urged not to change immediately, but to proceed slowly and cautiously toward a fully informed, considered decision regarding continuance of his or her self-critical practices.

Respond to Noncompliance

With clients who refuse to comply with the above directive, attempt one additional time to secure their compliance. Even if they again decline to continue their pathological self-critical practices, this additional refusal frequently solidifies the therapeutic gains inherent in doing so.

Respond to Compliance

With clients who implement the directive, (1) acknowledge and appreciate their efforts; (2) ask for a careful report on the nature of their self-critical behavior, its consequences, and other relevant observations; and (3) underscore any new sense of control over critic behaviors that the client reports. Use of this procedure, sometimes repeated once or twice in subsequent sessions, frequently results in clients achieving increased control over their pathological practices and making a decision to discontinue them.

Address Fears of Regression

Help clients who have successfully abandoned pathological self-critical practices to overcome common fears that a relapse will occur and that they will be helpless to prevent it. Do so by activities designed to reinforce further their sense of control over critic behaviors, thus minimizing their fears that a relapse could just "happen" to them. Having clients go over how they might arrange a deliberate relapse, actually prescribing such a relapse, and having them deliberately retain pathological critic behaviors "for special occasions" are some procedures for accomplishing this objective.

PROMOTING CONSTRUCTIVE MODES OF SELF-CRITICISM

Build On Clients' Existing Resources

Consistent with Milton Erickson's principle of "utilization" (O'Hanlon, 1987), observe a general policy of designing interventions that build on clients' existing competencies, understandings, values, and motivations.

Employ Two-Person Role Images

The principles of constructive self-criticism are essentially identical to the principles of constructive criticism of others. Many clients possess the latter, but have never thought to utilize them in their self-evaluative behavior. Therefore, when assessment reveals that they understand, value, and are skilled at roles such as parent, boss, teacher, or coach, this package of personal resources may be brought to bear in the service of constructive self-criticism. For example, the ability to be a good parent, which they possess, can become an excellent template for something they do not possess: the ability to be a competent self-critic.

Employ Concepts

Concepts such as "charity," "forgiveness," and "compassion" may be elucidated for many clients as constructive approaches to self-criticism. In doing so, however, it is imperative that they be operationalized in ways that clients can use. "Be charitable with yourself" is a useless suggestion for most people. "Select as a matter of personal policy those interpretations of situations that realistically portray you in the most positive light," is quite usable, especially with some guided practice, for many clients.

Encourage New Behavior

In the present approach, the paramount goal is that clients engage in new self-critical actions of a humane, effective, and constructive nature. To promote this, go beyond merely talking about such actions. Provide in-session opportunities for guided practice, give homework assignments, and in other ways promote active engagement in new critic behaviors.

ADDRESSING RESISTANCES AND OBSTACLES

Assess and Deal with Resistances

Clients fail to accept constructive self-critical perspectives and practices because they have various fears and reservations about doing so. They fear that the new self-critical practices will prove insufficiently motivating, will lead to them settling for mediocrity in their lives rather than excellence, will result in an unacceptable egotism, and more. The nature of such fears and reservations must be determined and the misconceptions on which they almost always rest subjected to cognitive modification procedures.

Assess and Deal with Obstacles

Some clients are restricted in their ability to change, not because of personal fears and reservations, but due to other kinds of obstacles. Significant persons in their lives may be so harshly and compellingly critical that some clients find it enormously difficult to adopt more constructive approaches to themselves. Other clients may "hang the hanging judge," thus unwittingly perpetuating the very problem they wish to stamp out. Yet others, given their historical self-degradations, may find new and more positive characterizations of themselves simply unthinkable. Again, such obstacles must be assessed, and ways found to help the client to overcome them.

THE THERAPEUTIC RELATIONSHIP

Make Accrediting Status Assignments

Assign statuses to clients that are accrediting, i.e., that convey eligibility to participate in the society in meaningful and fulfilling ways. Such statuses include one who is acceptable, who makes sense, whose best interests come first in this relationship, who is significant, who is an agent, and who has strengths. Assign these, not on the basis of empirical observation, but a priori. To the degree that one is able, view the client as a possessor of these statuses, and behave accordingly toward him or her. This may occur easily and naturally in many cases. In other more difficult ones, it may entail actively searching for more charitable perspectives on clients and/or correcting our own untoward reactions to them.

Maintain Therapist Eligibilities

Act in ways that enable the client to see you as a credible status assigner. Such ways include being honest, knowledgeable, competent, and willing to take authentic personal positions vis-à-vis the client. If disqualified by the client, engage in actions designed to recover lost status in his or her eyes.

Client Recognition

Act in ways that enhance the likelihood that status assignments made of the client are recognized by him or her. Do so especially under conditions where there is evidence that the client fails to perceive them.

Client Acceptance

Do whatever possible to see to it that assigned statuses are not only recognized, but accepted by the client. Explore barriers to such acceptance, and address them.

COMMITMENT

Encourage Commitment

Encourage clients to make deep, enduring personal commitments to constructive self-critical perspectives and practices. Use slogans and statements as devices to help them to maintain such commitments.

CONCLUSION

The goal of individuals becoming competent, constructive critics of themselves is of the utmost significance for their ability to lead full, satisfying, participatory lives. Possessed of such critic competencies, they become immeasurably more free to select and to carry out actions that are expressive of their genuine loves, interests, and values; and to do so unencumbered by damaged senses of elibibility, disabling emotional states, excessive concern with the reactions of others, and other impediments. It is the author's hope that the ideas contained in this book, which have been exceptionally helpful to him in securing such benefits for clients, will be of similar assistance to the reader.

REFERENCES

Abramson, L., Seligman, M. E. P., & Teasdale, J. (1978). Learned helplessness in humans: Critique and reformulation. *Journal of Abnormal Psychology, 87,* 32–48.

Arlow, J. A. (1989). Psychoanalysis. In R. Corsini & D. Wedding (Eds.), *Current psychotherapies* (4th ed.). Itasca, IL: Peacock.

Ashforth, S. J., & Cummings, I. I. (1983). Feedback as an individual resource. *Organizational Behavior and Human Performance, 32,* 370–398.

Assagioli, R. (1971). *Psychosynthesis.* Middlesex, England: Penguin Books.

Augustine (1955). *Augustine: Confessions and enchiridion* (Trans. A. Outler). In *The library of Christian classics* (Vol. 7). Philadelphia: Westminster Press.

Bandura, A. (1969). *Principles of behavior modification.* New York: Holt, Rinehart, & Winston.

Bandura, A. (1977). *Social learning theory.* Englewood Cliffs, NJ: Prentice-Hall.

Bandura, A. (1982). Self-efficacy beliefs in human agency. *American Psychologist, 37,* 122–147.

Bandura, A. (1986). *Social foundations of thought and action: A social cognitive theory.* Englewood Cliffs, NJ: Prentice-Hall.

Bandura, A. (1992). Exercise of personal agency through the self-efficacy mechanism. In R. Schwarzer (Ed.), *Self-efficacy: Thought and action.* Washington, DC: Hemisphere.

Baron, R. A. (1990). Countering the effects of destructive criticism: The relative effects of four interventions. *Journal of Applied Psychology, 75,* 235–245.

Barrow, J., & Moore, C. (1983). Group interventions with perfectionistic thinking. *The Personnel and Guidance Journal, 61,* 612–615.

Bateson, G., Jackson, D., Haley, J., & Weakland, J. (1956). Toward a theory of schizophrenia. *Behavioral Science, 1,* 251–264.

Baumrind, D. (1967). Child care patterns anteceding three patterns of preschool behavior. *Genetic Psychology Monographs, 75,* 43-88.

Baumrind, D. (1983). Rejoinder to Lewis's reinterpretation of parental firm control effects: Are authoritative families really harmonious? *Psychological Bulletin, 94,* 132–142.

Beck, A. (1976). *Cognitive therapy and the emotional disorders.* New York: Meridian.

Beck, A., & Emery, G. (1985). *Anxiety disorders and phobias.* New York: Basic Books.

Beck, A., & Weishaar, M. (1989). Cognitive therapy. In R. Corsini & D. Wedding (Eds.), *Current psychotherapies* (4th ed.). Itasca, IL: Peacock.

Beck, A., Rush, A., Shaw, B., & Emery, G. (1979). *Cognitive therapy of depression.* New York: Guilford.

Bennis, W. (1989). *On becoming a leader.* Reading, MA: Addison-Wesley.

Berglas, S., & Jones, E. E. (1978). Control of attributions about the self through self-handicapping strategies: The appeal of alcohol and the role of underachievement. *Personality and Social Psychology Bulletin, 4,* 200–206.

Bergner, R. (1981). The overseer regime: A descriptive and practical study of the obsessive-compulsive personality style. In K. Davis (Ed.), *Advances in descriptive psychology* (Vol. 1). Greenwich, CT: JAI Press.

Bergner, R. (1983). Emotions: A conceptual formulation and its clinical implications. In K. Davis & R. Bergner (Eds.), *Advances in descriptive psychology* (Vol. 3). Greenwich, CT: JAI Press.

Bergner, R. (1985). Paranoid style: A descriptive and pragmatic account. In K. Davis & T. Mitchell (Eds.), *Advances in descriptive psychology* (Vol. 4). Greenwich, CT: JAI Press.

Bergner, R. (1987). Undoing degradation. *Psychotherapy, 24,* 25–30.

Bergner, R. (1988). Status dynamic psychotherapy with depressed individuals. *Psychotherapy, 25,* 266–272.

Bergner, R. (1990). Father–daughter incest: Degradation and recovery from degradation. In T. Putman & K. Davis (Eds.), *Advances in descriptive psychology* (Vol. 5). Ann Arbor, MI: Descriptive Psychology Press.

Bergner, R. (1993). *Studies in psychopathology: The descriptive psychology approach.* Ann Arbor, MI: Descriptive Psychology Press.

Bergner, R. (1993). Victims into perpetrators. *Psychotherapy, 30,* 452–462.

Bergner, R., & Staggs, J. (1987). The positive therapeutic relationship as accreditation. *Psychotherapy, 24,* 315–320.

Berne, E. (1964). *Games people play.* New York: Grove Press.

Bowen, M. (1966). The use of family theory in clinical practice. *Comprehensive Psychiatry, 7,* 345–374.

Brady, J. (1980). Cited in M. Goldfried (Ed.), Some views of effective principles of psychotherapy. *Cognitive Therapy and Research, 4,* 271–306.

Brenner, C. (1974). An elementary textbook of psychoanalysis (rev. ed.). New York: Anchor Books.

Burns, D. (1980). Feeling good: The new mood therapy. New York: Morrow.

Burns, D., & Beck, A. (1978). Cognitive behavior modification of mood disorders. In J. Foreyt & D. Rathjen (Eds.), Cognitive behavior therapy: Research and application. New York: Plenum.

Camden, M. (1993). Forgiveness in therapy. Descriptive Psychology Bulletin, 22, 11–15.

Campbell, J., & Moyers, B. (1988). The power of myth. New York: Doubleday.

Carter, B., & McGoldrick, M. (1989). The changing family life cycle (2nd ed.). Needham Heights, MA: Allyn & Bacon.

Carver, C., & Scheier, M. (1990). Principles of self-regulation: Action and emotion. In E. Higgins & R. Sorrentino (Eds.), Handbook of motivation and cognition: Foundations of social behavior (Vol. 2). New York: Guilford.

Carver, C., & Scheier, M. (1992). Perspectives on personality. Needham Heights, MA: Allyn & Bacon.

Castaneda, C. (1968). The teachings of Don Juan: A Yaqui way of knowledge. Berkeley, CA: University of California Press.

Castaneda, C. (1972). A separate reality: Further conversations with Don Juan. New York: Pocket Books.

Castaneda, C. (1974). Journey to Ixtlan: The lessons of Don Juan. New York: Pocket Books.

Cervone, D. (1989). Effects of envisioning future activities on self-efficacy judgments and motivations: An availability heuristic interpretation. Cognitive Therapy and Research, 13, 247–261.

Cialdini, R. (1993). Influence: The psychology of persuasion (rev. ed.). New York: Quill/William Morrow.

Ciminero, A., Nelson, R., & Lipinski, D. (1977). Self-monitoring procedures. In A. Ciminero, K. Calhoun, & H. Adams (Eds.), Handbook of behavioral assessment. New York: John Wiley.

Cooley, C. (1902). Human nature and the social order. New York: Scribners.

Cramerus, M. (1990). Conflict, defense, and integration of self-presentations. Journal of Contemporary Psychotherapy, 20, 177–190.

Crow, T. J. (1989). A current view of the Type II syndrome: Age of onset, intellectual impairment, and the meaning of structural changes in the brain. British Journal of Psychiatry, 155, 15–20.

DePree, M. (1989). Leadership is an art. New York: Dell.

DeRubeis, R., & Beck, A. (1988). Cognitive therapy. In K. Dobson (Ed.), Handbook of cognitive–behavioral therapies. New York: Guilford.

DeShazer, S. (1984). The death of resistance. Family Process, 23, 11–21.

DeShazer, S. (1985). Keys to solution in brief therapy. New York: Basic Books.

DeShazer, S. (1988). Clues: Investigating solutions in brief therapy. New York: Basic Books.

Drew, E., & Connor, G. (1961). Discovering modern poetry. New York: Holt, Reinhart and Winston.

Driscoll, R. (1981). Self-criticism: Analysis and treatment. In K. Davis (Ed.), *Advances in descriptive psychology* (Vol. 1). Greenwich, CT: JAI Press.

Driscoll, R. (1984). *Pragmatic psychotherapy.* New York: Van Nostrand Reinhold.

Driscoll, R. (1989). Self-condemnation: A comprehensive framework for assessment and treatment. *Psychotherapy, 26,* 104–111.

Ellis, A. (1962). *Reason and emotion in psychotherapy.* New York: Lyle Stuart.

Ellis, A. (1984). Rational–emotive therapy. In R. Corsini (Ed.), *Current psychotherapies* (3rd ed.). Itasca, IL: Peacock.

Erickson, M. H. (1985). *Life reframing in hypnosis* (Vol. 2.). New York: Irvington.

Erikson, E. (1963). *Childhood and society* (2nd ed.). New York: Norton.

Farber, A. (1981). Castaneda's Don Juan as psychotherapist. In K. Davis (Ed.), *Advances in descriptive psychology* (Vol. 1). Greenwich, CT: JAI Press.

Fenichel, O. (1945). *The psychoanalytic theory of the neuroses.* New York: Norton.

Ferrari, J. (1992). Procrastinators and perfect behavior: An exploratory factor analysis of self-presentation, self-awareness, and self-handicapping components. *Journal of Research in Personality, 26,* 75–84.

Fisch, R., Weakland, J., & Segal, L. (1982). *The tactics of change: Doing therapy briefly.* San Francisco: Jossey-Bass.

Frank, J. (1963). *Persuasion and healing.* New York: Schocken Books.

Freud, S. (1917/1958). Mourning and melancholia. In J. Strachey (Ed.), *The complete psychological works of Sigmund Freud* (stand. ed., Vol. 14). London: Hogarth.

Freud, S. (1923). *The ego and the id.* (Trans. J. Riviere). London: Hogarth Press.

Frost, R., & Henderson, K. (1991). Perfectionism and reactions to athletic competition. *Journal of Sport and Exercise Psychology, 13,* 323–335.

Frost, R., Lahart, C, & Rosenblate, R. (1991). The development of perfectionism: A study of daughters and their parents. *Cognitive Therapy and Research, 15,* 469–489.

Fuller, B. (1985). Quoted in G. Seldes (Ed.), *The great thoughts.* New York: Ballantine.

Garfinkel, H. (1957). Conditions of successful degradation ceremonies. *American Journal of Sociology, 63,* 420–424.

Godfrey, D. K., Jones, E. E., & Lord, C. G. (1986). Self-promotion is not ingratiating. *Journal of Personality and Social Psychology, 50,* 106–115.

Goffman, E. (1959). *The presentation of self in everyday life.* New York: Doubleday Anchor.

Goffman, E. (1963). *Stigma: Notes on the management of spoiled identity.* Englewood Cliffs, NJ: Prentice-Hall.

Goldenberg, I., & Goldenberg, H. (1991). *Family therapy: An overview* (3rd ed.). Pacific Grove, CA: Brooks/Cole.

Greenberg, L., & Higgins, H. (1980). Effects of two-chair dialogues and focusing on conflict resolution. *Journal of Counseling Psychology, 27,* 221–224.

Grier, W., & Cobbs, P. (1968). *Black rage.* New York: Bantam Books.

Guidano, V. (1988). A systems, process-oriented approach to cognitive therapy. In K. Dobson (Ed.), *Handbook of cognitive–behavioral therapies.* New York: Guilford Press.

Haaga, D., & Beck, A. T. (1992). Cognitive therapy. In F. Paykel (Ed.), *Handbook of affective disorders* (2nd ed.). New York: Guilford.

Haley, J. (1980). *Leaving home: The therapy of disturbed young people.* New York: McGraw-Hill.

Hamachek, D. (1978). Psychodynamics of normal and neurotic perfectionism. *Psychology, 15,* 27–33.

Hardison, E. (1991). *Development of a comprehensive model of parenting: Six dimensions of parental responsibility.* Unpublished masters thesis, Illinois State University.

Harris, I., & Howard, K. (1984). Parental criticism and the adolescent experience. *Journal of Youth and Adolescence, 13,* 113–131.

Heider, F. (1958). *The psychology of interpersonal relations.* New York: Wiley.

Higgins, R. L., Snyder, C. R., & Berglas, S., (1990). *Self-handicapping: The paradox that isn't.* New York: Plenum.

Hoffman, L. (1981). *Foundations of family therapy.* New York: Basic Books.

Hoffman, M. (1984) Interaction of affect and cognition in empathy. In C. Izard, J. Kagan, & R. Zajonc (Eds.), *Emotions, cognition, and behavior.* Cambridge: Cambridge University Press.

Hoffman, M. (1988). Moral development. In M. Bornstein & M. Lamb (Eds.), *Developmental psychology: An advanced textbook.* Hillsdale, NJ: Erlbaum.

Jaenicke, C., Hammen, C., Zupan, B., Hiroto, D., Gordon, D., Adrian, C., & Burge, D. (1987). Cognitive vulnerability of children at risk for depression. *Journal of Abnormal Child Psychology, 15,* 559–572.

Jones, E. E., Farina, A., Hastorf, A. H., Markus, H., Miller, D. T., & Scott, R. A. (1984). *Social stigma: The psychology of marked relationships.* New York: W. H. Freeman.

Kahn, M. (1991). *Between therapist and client: The new relationship.* New York: W. H. Freeman.

Kanfer, F. (1970). Self-regulation: Research issues and speculations. In C. Neuringer & L. Michael (Eds.), *Behavior modification in clinical psychology.* New York: Appleton-Century-Crofts.

Kanfer, F. (1971). The maintenance of behavior by self-generated stimuli and reinforcements. In A. Jacobs & L. Sachs (Eds.), *The psychology of private events: Perspectives on covert response systems.* New York: Academic Press.

Kelly, G. (1955). *The psychology of personal constructs.* New York: Norton.

Kelly, W. (1984). Quoted in R. Driscoll, *Pragmatic psychotherapy*. New York: Van Nostrand Reinhold.

Kernberg, O. (1978). Why some people can't love. *Psychology Today*, June, 55–59.

Koestner, R., Zuroff, D., & Powers, T. (1991). Family origins of adolescent self-criticism and its continuity into adulthood. *Journal of Abnormal Psychology*, 100, 191–197.

Kohut, H. (1971). *The analysis of the self*. New York: International Universities Press.

Kohut, H. (1977). *The restoration of the self*. New York: International Universities Press.

Kuczynski, L., Zahn-Waxler, C., & Radke-Yarrow, M. (1987). Development and content of imitation in the second and third year of life: A socialization perspective. *Developmental Psychology*, 23, 276–282.

Laing, R. D. (1965). *The divided self*. Baltimore: Penguin.

Lang, P., Melamed, B., & Hart, J. (1970). A psychophysiological analysis of fear modification using an automated desensitization procedure. *Journal of Abnormal Psychology*, 76, 220–234.

Lange, A., & Jakubowski, P. (1976). *Responsible assertive behavior*. Champaign, IL: Research Press.

Lazarus, A. (1980). Cited in M. Goldfried (Ed.), Some views of effective principles of psychotherapy. *Cognitive Therapy and Research*, 4, 271–306.

Lazarus, R., (1966). *Psychological stress and the coping process*. New York: McGraw-Hill.

Lazarus, R., & Folkman, S. (1984). *Stress, appraisal, and coping*. New York: Springer.

Liberman, P. (1969). Behavioral approaches to family and couple therapy. *American Journal of Orthopsychiatry*. 39, 86–94.

Liebert, R., & Spiegler, M. (1994). *Personality: Strategies and issues* (7th ed.). Pacific Grove, CA: Brooks/Cole.

Maccoby, E., & Martin, J. (1983). Socialization in the context of the family: Parent–child interaction. In E. M. Hetherington (Ed.), *Handbook of child psychology: Vol. 4. Socialization, personality, and personal development* (4th ed.). New York: Wiley.

Marshall, K. (1991). A bulimic life pattern. In M. Roberts & R. Bergner (Eds.), *Clinical topics: Adolescent–family problems, bulimia, chronic mental illness, and mania*. Ann Arbor, MI: Descriptive Psychology Press.

McKay, J. (1992). Building self-esteem in children. In M. McKay & P. Fanning, *Self-esteem* (2nd ed.). Oakland, CA: New Harbinger Publications.

McKay, M., & Fanning, P. (1992). *Self-esteem* (2nd ed.). Oakland, CA: New Harbinger Publications.

Mead, G. (1934). *Mind, self, & society*. Chicago: University of Chicago Press.

Meichenbaum, D. (1973). *Cognitive behavior modification*. New York: Plenum.

Mizer, J. E. (1964). Cipher in the snow. *National Educational Association Journal*, 53, 8–10.

Niebuhr, R. (1956). *An interpretation of Christian ethics.* New York: Meridian.

Nolen-Hoeksema, S., Girgus, J., & Seligman, M. (1987). Learned helplessness in children: A longitudinal study of depression, achievement, and explanatory style. *Journal of Personality and Social Psychology, 51,* 435–442.

O'Hanlon, W. H. (1987). *Taproots: Underlying principles of Milton Erickson's therapy and hypnosis.* New York: Norton.

Ohbuchi, K., Kameda, M., & Agarie, N. (1989). Apology as aggression control: Its role in mediating appraisal of and response to harm. *Journal of Personality and Social Psychology, 56,* 219–227.

Ossorio, P. G. (1976) *Clinical topics* (LRI Report #11). Whittier and Boulder: Linguistic Research Institute.

Ossorio, P. G. (1978). *What actually happens.* Columbia: University of South Carolina Press.

Ossorio, P. G. (1981) An outline of descriptive psychology. In K. Davis (Ed.), *Advances in descriptive psychology* (Vol. 1). Greenwich, CT: JAI Press.

Ossorio, P. G. (1982). *Place* (LRI Report #30a). Boulder, CO: Linguistic Research Institute.

Ossorio, P. G. (1985). Pathology. In K. Davis & T. Mitchell (Eds.), *Advances in descriptive psychology* (Vol. 4). Greenwich, CT: JAI Press.

Ossorio, P. G. (1990). Appraisal. In A. Putman & K. Davis (Eds.), *Advances in descriptive psychology* (Vol. 5). Ann Arbor, MI: Descriptive Psychology Press.

Ossorio, P., & Sternberg, K. (1981). *Status management: A theory of punishment and rehabilitation* (LRI Report #25). Boulder, CO: Linguistic Research Institute.

Paine, S., Radicchi, J., Rosellini, L., Deutchman, L., & Darch, C. (1983). *Structuring your classroom for academic success.* Champaign, Il: Research Press.

Perls, F., Hefferline, R., & Goodman, P. (1951). *Gestalt therapy.* New York: Dell Publishing.

Peterson, C., Maier, S. F., & Seligman, M. E. P. (1993). *Learned helplessness: A theory for the age of personal control.* New York: Oxford University Press.

Pervin, L. (1983). The stasis and flow of behavior: Toward a theory of goals. In M. Page & R. Dienstbier (Eds.), *Nebraska symposium on motivation* (Vol. 31). Lincoln: University of Nebraska Press.

Powers, T., & Zuroff, D. (1988). Interpersonal consequences of overt self-criticism: A comparison with neutral and self-enhancing presentations of self. *Journal of Personality and Social Psychology, 4,* 1054–1062.

Pryor, J. B., & Reeder, G. D. (1993). Collective and individual representations of HIV/AIDS stigma. In J. Pryor & G. Reeder (Eds.), *The social psychology of HIV infection.* Hillsdale, NJ: Erlbaum.

Putman, A. (1990). Organizations. In A. Putman & K. Davis (Eds.), *Advances in descriptive psychology* (Vol. 5). Ann Arbor, MI: Descriptive Psychology Press.

Rado, S. (1929). The problem of melancholia. *International Journal of Psycho-Analysis, 9,* 420–438.

Raimy, V. (1975). *Misconceptions of the self.* San Francisco: Jossey-Bass.

Raskin, N., & Rogers, C. (1989). Person-centered therapy. In R. Corsinsi & D. Wedding (Eds.), *Current psychotherapies* (4th ed.). Itasca, IL: Peacock.

Reeder, G., & Fulks, J. (1980). When actions speak louder than words: Implicational schemata and the attribution of ability. *Journal of Experimental Social Psychology, 16,* 33–46.

Rehm, L. (1977). A self-control model of depression. *Behavior Therapy, 8,* 787–804.

Rehm, L., & Rokke, P. (1988). Self-management therapies. In K. Dobson (Ed.), *Handbook of cognitive–behavior therapies.* New York: Guilford.

Roberts, M. (1985). I and thou: A study of personal relationships. In K. Davis & T. Mitchell (Eds.), *Advances in descriptive psychology* (Vol. 4). Greenwich, CT: JAI Press.

Rogers, C. (1951). *Client-centered therapy.* Boston: Houghton-Mifflin.

Rogers, C. (1957). The necessary and sufficient conditions of therapeutic personality change. *Journal of Consulting Psychology, 21,* 95–103.

Rogers, C. (1959). A theory of therapy, personality, and interpersonal relations. In S. Koch (Ed.), *Psychology: A study of a science* (Vol. 3). New York: McGraw-Hill.

Rosenthal, R. (1974). *On the social psychology of the self-fulfilling prophecy: Further evidence for Pygmalion effects and their mediating mechanisms.* New York: MSS Modular Publications.

Rubin, T. I. (1975). *Compassion and self-hate.* New York: Collier.

Schwartz, W. (1979). Degradation, accreditation, and rites of passage. *Psychiatry, 42,* 138–146.

Schwarzer, R. (1992). Self-efficacy in the adoption and maintenance of health behaviors: Theoretical approaches and a new model. In R. Schwarzer (Ed.), *Self-efficacy: Thought control of action.* Washington, DC: Hemisphere.

Segal, L. (1991). Brief family therapy. In A. Horne & J. Passmore (Eds.), *Family counselling and therapy.* Itasca, IL: Peacock.

Selvini-Palazzoli, M., Boscolo, L, Cecchin, G., & Prata, G. (1978). *Paradox and counterparadox.* New York: Jason Aronson.

Selvini-Palazzoli, M., Cirillo, S., Selvini, M., & Sorrentino, A. M., (1989). *Family games: General models of psychotic processes in the family.* New York: Norton.

Shapiro, D. (1965). *Neurotic styles.* New York: Basic Books.

Shideler, M. (1988). *Persons, behavior, and the world.* New York: University Press of America.

Shoobs, N. (1964). Role playing in the individual psychotherapy interview. *Journal of Individual Psychology, 20,* 84–89.

Snyder, C. R., & Higgins, R. L. (1988). Excuses: Their effective role in the negotiation of reality. *Psychological Bulletin, 104,* 23–35.

Snyder, C. R., & Smith, T. W. (1982). Symptoms as self-handicapping strategies. In G. Weary & H. L. Mirels (Eds.), *Integrations of clinical and social psychology.* New York: Oxford University Press.

Snyder, C. R., Higgins, R. L., & Stucky, R. J. (1983). *Excuses: Masquerades in search of grace.* New York: Wiley/Interscience.

Sorotzkin, B. (1985). The quest for perfection: Avoiding guilt or avoiding shame? *Psychotherapy, 22,* 564–571.

Stephan, S., & Stephan, S. (1990). *Two social psychologies.* Belmont, CA: Wadsworth.

Stone, H., & Stone, S. (1993). *Embracing your inner critic.* San Francisco: Harper Collins.

Sweet, A. (1984). The therapeutic relationship in behavior therapy. *Clinical Psychology Review, 4,* 253–272.

Uleman, J., & Bargh, J. (1989). *Unintended thought.* New York: Guilford.

Vygotsky, L. (1962). *Thought and language.* Cambridge, MA: MIT Press. (Original work published 1934)

Watts, A. (1940). *The meaning of happiness.* New York: Harper & Row.

Watzlawick, P. (1978). *The language of change.* New York: Basic Books.

Watzlawick, P. (1988). *Ultra-solutions.* New York: Norton.

Watzlawick, P., Weakland, J., & Fisch, R. (1974). *Change: Principles of problem formation and problem resolution.* New York: Norton.

Webster's II New Riverside University Dictionary (1985). Boston: Houghton Mifflin.

Wechsler, R. (1993). Personality and manic states: A status dynamic formulation of manic disorder. In R. Bergner (Ed.), *Studies in psychopathology: The descriptive psychology approach.* Ann Arbor, MI: Descriptive Psychology Press.

Weeks, G., & L'Abate, L. (1982). *Paradoxical psychotherapy: Theory and practice with individuals, couples, and families.* New York: Brunner-Mazel.

Wegner, D. (1989). *White bears and other unwanted thoughts: Suppression, obsession, and the psychology of mental control.* New York: Viking Press.

Wheeler, L., & Miyake, K. (1992). Social comparison in everyday life. *Journal of Personality and Social Psychology, 62,* 760–773.

White, D. (1988). Taming the critic: The use of imagery with clients who procrastinate. *Journal of Mental Imagery, 12,* 125–133.

Wills, T. A. (1986). Discussion remarks on social comparison theory. *Personality and Social Psychology Bulletin, 12,* 282–288.

Wilson, G. (1989). Behavior therapy. In R. Corsini & D. Wedding (Eds.), *Current psychotherapies* (4th ed.). Itasca, Ill.: F. E. Peacock.

INDEX